Heart Disease
and High Cholesterol

Beating the Odds

Heart Disease and High Cholesterol

Beating the Odds

C. Richard Conti, M.D., F.A.C.C.,
and Diana Tonnessen

Illustrations by Mona Mark

Addison-Wesley Publishing Company

Reading, Massachusetts · Menlo Park, California · New York
Don Mills, Ontario · Wokingham, England · Amsterdam
Bonn · Sydney · Singapore · Tokyo · Madrid · San Juan
Paris · Seoul · Milan · Mexico City · Taipei

Figure 3, Blood Cholesterol and Your Risk of Coronary Heart Disease, reprinted with permission from: Martin, M.J., Hulley, S.B., Browner, W.S., Kuller, L.H., and Wentworth, D. "Serum Cholesterol, Blood Pressure, and Mortality: Implications from a Cohort of 361,622 Men." *The Lancet,* vol. 2, no. 8513, pp. 933–936. Copyright by The Lancet, Ltd. 1986.

The RISKO self-assessment test is reproduced with permission, copyright RISKO, 1985, by American Heart Association.

Figure 5, the graph entitled Danger of Heart Attack by Risk Factors Present from the *1991 Heart and Stroke Facts* (#55-0379), copyright 1990, American Heart Association, reproduced with permission.

The 1983 Height and Weight Tables reprinted by courtesy of the Metropolitan Life Insurance Company.

Instructions for the Relaxation Response, which appear on page 84, are adapted from Dr. Herbert Benson's book *The Relaxation Response* (copyright 1975 by William Morrow and Company, Inc.) and are used with the permission of William Morrow and Company, Inc., Publishers, New York.

Library of Congress Cataloging-in-Publication Data

Conti, C. Richard (Charles Richard), 1934–
    Heart disease and high cholesterol : beating the odds
    C. Richard Conti and Diana Tonnessen : illustrations by Mona Mark.
    p.   cm. — (Reducing your hereditary risk)
Includes bibliographical references and index.
    ISBN 0-201-57782-8
    1. Heart—Diseases—Prevention. 2. Hypercholesteremia–
–Prevention. I. Tonnessen, Diana. II. Title.
RC672.C62 1992
616.1'205—dc20   91-44003
                                              CIP

Cover design by Martucci Studio
Text design by Joyce C. Weston
Set in 10-point Clarendon Light by NK Graphics, Keene, NH

2 3 4 5 6 7 8 9–MU–9695949392
Second printing, November 1992

Contents

List of Illustrations

CHAPTER

1

How Heart Disease Runs in the Family

PEOPLE tend to think of genetic illness as something they're helpless to do anything about, that if a disease is "in their genes," their fate is somehow sealed. So it may be more than a little unsettling to learn that coronary heart disease—the leading cause of death in America today—is hereditary. In fact, coronary heart disease may be one of the most common inherited illnesses.

This fact may be especially disconcerting when heart disease hits close to home: Someone in your own family—a parent, grandparent, or sibling—suffers a heart attack or is diagnosed with coronary heart disease before age 50. After the crisis has passed and the initial shock has worn off, you may begin to feel a little more vulnerable yourself. You may start to wonder, too, if there are steps you can take to protect yourself and other family members from a similar fate.

Take heart. Physicians and researchers now know that what you've inherited is a *genetic predisposition* to heart disease that can be triggered by such life-style factors as your diet. And thanks to research on cardiovascular disease over the last 20 years, they know more than ever about what those influences are. Most of them—your diet, activity level, cigarette smoking, even the way you respond to stress—are things you have direct control over. In effect, then, one of the most prevalent hereditary illnesses may also be one of the most highly preventable.

There's more reason for optimism. The same genetic research that tells the medical community that heart attacks are hereditary is leading to more specific diagnostic tests that can target those at greatest risk. And since heart disease is a slowly progressing illness that develops over a lifetime, the sooner you know you're at risk, the better your chances are of beating the odds.

There's hope, too, that a current project to map the 50,000 to 100,000 genes that make up the human body will eventually lead to a cure for heart disease. So far, geneticists involved with the Human Genome Project have identified only about 2,000 of the genes that make us uniquely human. But they've cataloged close to 5,000 inherited conditions that can occur even if one out of 100,000 genes carries a defect. In the last few years new technology has stepped up progress on the Human Genome Project, and researchers are feverishly adding more pieces to the puzzle every week.

Once medical specialists know the genetic codes for healthy people, they can start to pinpoint even more genetic defects that lead to illness. With a better understanding of what causes an illness, more effective treatments and preventive measures can be developed. The most exciting news yet: the first human experiments to use gene therapy are already under way and include work on a genetic treatment for people with an inherited form of high cholesterol. (We'll talk more about these experiments in chapter 10.) If the experiments are successful, they promise to revolutionize the way physicians practice medicine. The research and experiments will have a profound effect on the way they treat (and prevent) heart disease, too, because as you're about to learn, many of the predisposing factors for heart disease are being traced back to genetic roots.

To understand how heart attacks can be hereditary, it helps to know a little about your heart and how heart disease develops. Your heart, a muscle a little larger than your fist, pumps some 2,000 gallons of blood through your body in a day. The circulating blood carries oxygen and nutrients through a vast network of blood vessels to all organs and tissues—including the heart itself. Your circulatory system also carries waste products from the cells back to the liver, kidneys, and lungs for processing and disposal. There are several different types of diseases of the heart and blood vessels, collectively known as *cardiovascular disease.* High blood pressure, coronary heart disease, and stroke (a disruption in blood flow to the brain caused by a blood clot or broken blood vessel) are the major types of cardiovascular disease.

The leading cause of heart attacks is *coronary heart disease,* which is what we'll be discussing in this book. Coronary heart disease occurs when deposits of fat and scar tissue, or *plaques,* gradually build up on the inner walls of the blood vessels (fig. 1). No one is sure exactly why these plaques develop. Some researchers think that the innermost lining of the blood vessel wall somehow becomes damaged, allowing fat, calcium, and other deposits to build up. For reasons not yet clear, plaques most often accumulate on the coronary arteries—the blood vessels that supply nutrients and oxygen to the heart muscle.

Over time (usually several decades), the plaques begin to narrow the blood vessels, a process called *atherosclerosis.* As the coronary arteries narrow, the blood supply to the heart is gradually reduced. Most people adjust to this reduced blood supply over the years. The only sign of trouble may be chest pain during strenuous activity, or *angina pectoris,* stemming from the lack of oxygen and nutrients to

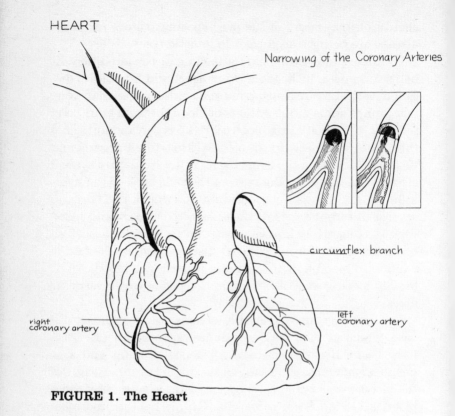

HEART

Narrowing of the Coronary Arteries

circumflex branch

left
coronary artery

right
coronary artery

FIGURE 1. The Heart

the heart. The pain subsides after a few moments of rest because a resting heart doesn't need as much blood as an active one.

A heart attack occurs when enough plaques accumulate to produce complete blockage of a coronary artery. Or a blood clot (*coronary thrombosis*) may form on a smaller plaque and choke off the blood supply to the heart. With no oxygen or nutrients, the heart tissue supplied by the blocked artery begins to die.

Physicians have known for some time that people who develop coronary heart disease often have abnormally high levels of a fatty substance called *cholesterol* circulating in their blood. You've probably heard and read a lot about cholesterol, most of it bad news, over the past few years—for instance, that cholesterol is one of the main components of artery-clogging plaques and that the more cholesterol you have in your bloodstream, the more likely you are to develop these plaques and possibly suffer a heart attack.

However, you need a certain amount of cholesterol to survive. In fact, every cell in your body contains cholesterol, which is used to form cell membranes that help carry out the cell's basic functions. Cholesterol also helps manufacture certain hormones. Cholesterol in your skin acts as a barrier to keep vital body fluids in and harmful substances out. Indeed, cholesterol is so important to your health and well-being that *your body is genetically programmed to manufacture most of the cholesterol it needs.*

What the new research has uncovered are flaws in the genetic controls for cholesterol (and other fats, or *lipids,* circulating in your bloodstream) that appear to cause elevated cholesterol levels and, in turn, put some people at increased risk of heart disease. (Researchers are also finding that certain genetic defects actually *protect* some people from developing heart disease.) Before we talk about what can go wrong with the genetic codes for cholesterol, let's take a look at how a healthy person manufactures and processes it.

Your body has a sophisticated system of checks and balances—a cholesterol thermostat, of sorts—to ensure that each of your 75 billion cells gets the cholesterol it needs to survive. The master controls for this thermostat reside in the liver, which makes most of the cholesterol your body needs. The liver also processes dietary fat and cholesterol in the foods you eat (found chiefly in meats and dairy products), which, as you'll see later on, can affect the levels of cholesterol circulating in your bloodstream.

Like all fats, cholesterol doesn't dissolve in water—the main component of blood. For this reason, the liver packages cholesterol into protein carriers called *lipoproteins.* The protein part of the lipoprotein allows the fat molecule to circulate in the bloodstream.

There are several different types of lipoproteins, each of which plays a role in the processing and handling of cholesterol—and in influencing your risk of coronary heart disease. *Low-density lipoproteins* (LDL cholesterol) deliver cholesterol to virtually every cell in your body and help deposit it there. Any excess LDL cholesterol is returned to the liver, where it is broken down and cleared from the body. Excessive amounts of LDL cholesterol in the bloodstream may be deposited in the artery walls, which is how LDL cholesterol became known as the "bad" cholesterol. *High-density lipoproteins* (HDL cholesterol), manufactured in the small intestine and the liver and released into the bloodstream, haul cholesterol back to the liver for processing and disposal. HDL cholesterol may even help remove cholesterol deposits from the artery walls, which is why it is often called the "good" cholesterol.

Several studies now suggest that the protein components of lipoproteins, or *apolipoproteins,* may better predict heart disease risk than LDL and HDL cholesterol. Scientists have identified several types of apolipoproteins (also called "apo's"), which go by the names apolipoproteins A, B, C, E, and (a).

Triglycerides, fat molecules manufactured by the liver and also derived from fat in the foods you eat, may play a role in the development of heart disease, too. Triglycerides are mainly a source of energy for the body. However, high blood levels of triglycerides appear to increase the risk of heart disease for some people.

Very low density lipoproteins, which can be thought of as precursors of LDL cholesterol, contain both cholesterol and triglycerides. Their chief job is to transport triglycerides to the body's muscles and fat tissues to be used (or stored) as energy. Once the triglycerides have been delivered, the lipoprotein, now containing mostly cholesterol, becomes an LDL particle.

Certain types of *receptors* may also influence your risk of developing heart disease. In simplest terms, receptors are specialized parts of the cell, located on the cell's surface, that act like magnets to attract and bind various substances to the cell.

There are many different kinds of receptors in your body. The important ones for the purposes of our discussion are receptors that help regulate the processing of cholesterol and fat in your body. Perhaps the best known of these are *LDL receptors,* which bind LDL cholesterol to the cell so it can be deposited into the cell wall. All of your body's cells contain LDL receptors, but most of the LDL receptors in your body reside in the liver, where their chief role is to clear excess LDL cholesterol from the bloodstream and absorb it back into the liver.

In a healthy person, the liver, the various lipoproteins, and receptors work in concert to meet and not exceed the body's cholesterol needs. However, certain genetic flaws may throw off this system's balance, resulting in abnormally high levels of cholesterol.

The genetic condition most well known by the medical establishment goes by the tongue-twisting name *familial hypercholesterolemia* (FH), caused by a flaw in the gene that controls the production of LDL receptors. About one in 500 people is affected, making this the most common simple hereditary illness. Most affected people have *heterozygous FH,* meaning that they inherited a copy of the defective gene from only one of their parents (fig. 2). People with heterozygous FH have about half the number of LDL receptors as unaffected people, and cholesterol levels about twice as high. If left untreated, affected men risk suffering a first heart attack in their thirties and forties, while affected women may suffer a first heart attack in their fifties. About one in a million people inherits a defective gene from *both*

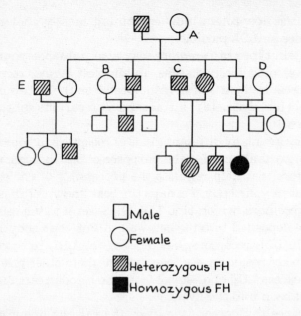

☐ Male
◯ Female
▨ Heterozygous FH
■ Homozygous FH

FIGURE 2. How High Blood Cholesterol Runs in the Family. *Familial hypercholesterolemia is an autosomal dominant trait, meaning that only one defective gene needs to be inherited for a person to develop the condition. (A recessive trait, such as blue eyes, requires two copies of a gene—one from each parent—to be expressed.) If only one parent has FH (A and B), each child born to that parent has a 50/50 chance of inheriting the defective gene and developing heterozygous FH. In the unlikely event that both parents have heterozygous FH (C), there's a one-in-four chance that a child will be born healthy, a 50/50 chance that the child will inherit one copy of the defective gene, and a one-in-four chance that the child will inherit the lethal combination of two defective genes, or homozygous FH. Children who don't inherit the defective gene (D), don't have to worry about passing it along to their children—unless, of course, they marry someone with FH (E).*

parents and develops a much more serious form of the disease, called *homozygous FH.* These people have few or no LDL receptors, and cholesterol levels about four times higher than those of unaffected people. People with homozygous FH usually suffer their first heart attack in their teens.

Fortunately, as you'll see in the pages to come, the outlook for treating the condition is better than ever. Changes in diet alone often suffice to lower blood cholesterol to safer levels among heterozygotes. Several cholesterol-lowering drugs are now available for stubborn cases, as well. And although homozygotes generally don't respond to diet or drug therapies, they sometimes are helped by liver transplants, made possible through advanced technology and immunosuppressive drugs that prevent organ rejection. Human experiments involving a new type of gene therapy for people with homozygous FH are now being planned (see ch. 10). If the experiments succeed, the researchers hope the treatment will lower cholesterol in affected people by up to 50 percent.

Familial hypercholesterolemia explains why one in 500 people has high blood cholesterol levels, but the genetic disorder doesn't begin to account for the high blood cholesterol of an estimated 47 million Americans. These people, who are said to have *primary (nonfamilial) hypercholesterolemia,* are at no less risk of developing coronary heart disease than people with FH. And while the medical term suggests that the problem isn't inherited, an increasing number of researchers now suspect that genetic factors— perhaps several of them combined—somehow make these people more susceptible to outside influences on cholesterol, such as diet. A diet high in saturated fats, cholesterol, and calories (like the typical Euro-American diet) may raise LDL cholesterol to "high-risk" levels in people who wouldn't otherwise have high cholesterol. Genetic factors would also help explain why many people who eat the same high-fat, high-cholesterol foods *don't* develop dangerously high blood cholesterol levels.

New research is zeroing in on genetic defects in the various apolipoproteins that may increase a person's susceptibility to heart disease. Scientists have already identified a genetic defect of the apo B protein carrier that helps transport LDL cholesterol through the body. Affected people have high levels of LDL cholesterol even though they have normal LDL receptors. Other genetic flaws affecting apolipoproteins A and C result in low levels of the heart-protective HDL cholesterol and subsequent premature heart disease.

Genes also appear to influence blood levels of lipoprotein (a), or *Lp(a),* which many researchers refer to as "L-p-little a," a recently discovered fat particle that's receiving increasing attention these days for its role in the development of heart disease. Several studies have now linked high levels of Lp(a) with an increased risk of heart attack. The problem with Lp(a) is that it is practically a chemical twin to a clot-dissolving substance in the blood called *plasminogen.* We suspect that Lp(a) somehow takes the place of plasminogen in the artery wall and short-circuits the blood vessel's natural ability to dissolve clots, increasing the risk that a blood clot may form. And a blood clot that gets lodged in a coronary artery can trigger a heart attack.

We suspect genes may also precipitate several other conditions that increase a person's risk of heart disease, particularly hypertension, diabetes, and obesity.

Some 58 million Americans have *hypertension,* elevated blood pressure levels that are considered a major risk factor for heart attacks. Scientists have suspected for some time now that the condition has a hereditary component. Many researchers have speculated that blacks develop high blood pressure much more frequently than whites because of a genetic predisposition.

Scientists at Boston University School of Medicine have now pinpointed a tiny genetic defect believed to be at least partly responsible for "sodium-sensitive" high blood pressure in a strain of rats prone to hypertension. Rats with the defect develop high blood pressure when fed high-salt diets; the animals without the defect do not. The researchers suspect a similar genetic error may be present in humans, which may help explain why one-third to one-half of people with hypertension are sodium-sensitive in terms of blood pressure.

Another risk factor for heart disease, *diabetes mellitus,* also appears to be hereditary. Diabetes is marked by abnormally high blood sugar levels caused when the body either doesn't produce enough insulin or doesn't use insulin efficiently. Diabetes occurs in two major forms: insulin-dependent (Type I) and non-insulin-dependent (Type II) diabetes. Non-insulin-dependent diabetes is much more common and, overall, contributes more to coronary heart disease than does insulin-dependent diabetes. Although no specific genes or genetic markers have been identified for either Type I or Type II diabetes, both conditions are believed to be inherited. Some studies suggest that non-insulin dependent diabetes is related to a hereditary predisposition that may be triggered by obesity, severe stress, pregnancy, or other factors.

Obesity, yet another risk factor for heart disease, also seems to run in the family. Researchers have already found that the body mass index (a measure of body fat) of adopted children more closely resembles that of their biological parents and siblings than that of their adoptive parents. And in a major study comparing the body mass index of identical twins reared in separate homes, researchers at the University of Pennsylvania in Philadelphia found that 70 percent of the twins shared a similar body mass index. Clearly, your genes play a major role in determining your weight as an adult.

This is not to say, however, that you're a slave to your genes. In fact, you can control most of the inherited conditions we've talked about so far; your risk of coronary heart disease can be substantially reduced through changes in life-style habits that you can make yourself. Right now. Starting today.

Dramatic new evidence now suggests that narrowing of the arteries *can be reversed* by eating a very low-fat diet and making other changes in life-style habits. In a preliminary study conducted by Dr. Dean Ornish at the University of California at San Francisco, men and women with coronary artery disease ate a vegetarian diet consisting of less than 10 percent fat, exercised moderately every day, and practiced yoga and meditation for an hour a day. Cholesterol levels of the volunteers dropped from an average 227 milligrams per deciliter (mg/dl) to 136 mg/dl. (Cholesterol levels less than 200 mg/dl are considered "desirable.") More important, *angiographies* (in which a fluid is injected into the blood and X rays are taken to reveal the amount of blockage in the coronary arteries) showed a measurable widening of the coronary arteries among the people who continued the strict regimen for a year. More research must be conducted before we'll know with certainty just how effective life-style changes are at reversing atherosclerosis. But so far, the results appear promising.

Reducing blood pressure also reduces the risk of heart disease. The largest study to date found that for every five- to six-point fall in blood pressure, there's a 20 to 25 percent decline in the risk of heart disease (and a 30 to 40 percent drop in the risk of stroke). Although the people in this study were given drugs to lower their blood pressure, other research has shown that diet and exercise alone are often enough to lower mildly elevated blood pressure (the kind most people have) to normal levels.

Physicians have known for a while now that many people with non-insulin dependent diabetes can control it by losing weight and watching what they eat. Even people who appear to have inherited their parents' "fat genes" aren't necessarily resigned to a lifetime of obesity. While obesity may be up to 70 percent nature, several studies have shown that nurture (specifically, diet and exercise) is important, too.

Although awareness of your genetic makeup may discourage you, knowing that you may be at somewhat greater risk of heart disease puts you ahead of the game. Your knowledge allows you to alter your life-style habits now, before the disease progresses too far. In fact, a positive, take-charge attitude may be the best protection you have. Numerous studies have suggested that, in general, people with a positive attitude who take an active role in the management of a disease fare better than those who feel resigned to an unchangeable fate and act accordingly.

In the pages that follow, you'll learn how you can help keep an inherited predisposition to heart disease from becoming a grim reality. But first, let's take a look at just how "at risk" you are.

CHAPTER
2

Gauging Your Risk

O NE of the many promises genetic research holds is the ability to more accurately predict—and minimize—a person's future risk of illness through genetic testing. Already, this kind of testing has become commonplace during early pregnancy—newborns are now screened for up to nine inherited disorders. In the not-too-distant future, it may be possible to take a simple blood test and learn within hours or days whether a heart attack is likely in your future—or whether you're in the clear.

Of course, discovering that a heart attack may be hidden in your genes can be a frightening proposition. Remember, though, that knowing you may be at risk years or even decades in advance of any symptoms gives you that much more time to take action and improve your odds of *not* having a heart attack.

Scientists are making significant inroads toward developing just such a genetic screening test for heart disease. Researchers have already located the gene suspected of causing familial hypercholesterolemia on the short arm of chromosome 19. They also have pinpointed many of the genes governing the various apolipoproteins. The genes for apo E, C-I, and C-II, for instance, are all on chromosome 19. Chromosome 6 contains the genetic controls for apo (a). And apo A-I and C-III are controlled by genes on chromosome 11.

However, researchers still have a long way to go. A major stumbling block: even after a suspected gene has been located, there may be a variety of mutations within a single gene that cause the same disorder. For instance, there are some 60 to 100 different mutations within the gene that causes *cystic fibrosis,* the most common fatal genetic disease of young Americans. However, since only one of those mutations causes about 70 percent of all cases, scientists have been able to develop a test that can now detect roughly three-quarters of all adults who risk having children with cystic fibrosis.

At this point, at least 16 different mutations have been found to cause the LDL-receptor defects of FH, making the development of a mass screening test for FH a little too complex. (Genetic tests to screen for conditions involving more than one gene—as researchers suspect may be the case with other types of high blood cholesterol, high blood pressure, diabetes, and obesity—are more complicated still.) However, families who are suspected of having FH can undergo DNA testing. A small amount of blood is taken from each family member and sent to a laboratory, where the genetic material DNA (*deoxyribonucleic acid*) is analyzed. Geneticists look for mutations within the FH gene on chromosome 19 that are common to members of that particular family. In this way, they can determine which individuals are affected long before symptoms of heart disease appear. Prenatal tests can also be performed to detect whether a fetus is affected.

In the near future, diagnostic tests with more mass appeal will measure blood levels of certain apolipoproteins. Studies have already shown that elevated levels of Lp(a) indicate a strongly increased risk for coronary heart disease among people with FH. For now, however, the tests are too complicated and too costly to be of practical value.

Even if a mass screening test for heart disease were developed, it wouldn't be 100 percent accurate. The test would indicate only whether you do or do not carry a certain genetic defect. Rarely can these tests reveal how severely you would be affected, nor can they predict when or if symptoms would appear. But the tests give us more information to make an educated guess about a person's odds of developing heart disease later in life.

EARLY WARNING SIGNS

The first step in gauging your risk of heart disease is to familiarize yourself with a few early warning signs:

Family history: Your family tree and family medical history can reveal important clues about your own chances of developing heart disease. If one of your parents has a genetic predisposition to heart disease, the odds are 50/50 that you do too. You may be at greater risk if

- Your father or a brother suffers angina (chest pain), a heart attack, or sudden death before age 55, *or* your mother or a sister develops heart disease before age 60.
- Your parents, brothers, or sisters have elevated cholesterol levels (total cholesterol above 240 mg/dl of blood; elevated LDL cholesterol or triglycerides; or low levels of HDL cholesterol).
- A parent or sibling has high blood pressure or diabetes.

Elevated blood cholesterol levels: Your own blood cholesterol levels are another barometer of your risk of developing coronary heart disease. People with blood cholesterol levels of 240 mg/dl or greater have more than twice the risk of someone whose cholesterol is 200 mg/dl (fig. 3). Your doctor

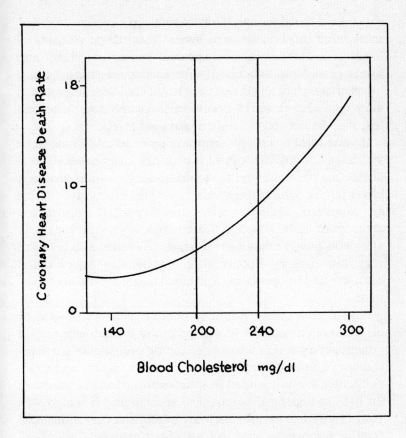

FIGURE 3. Blood Cholesterol and Your Risk of Coronary Heart Disease. *As blood cholesterol levels rise, so does your risk of developing coronary heart disease. If your blood cholesterol level is 240 mg/dl or greater, you are more than twice as likely to develop heart disease as someone whose cholesterol level is 200 mg/dl. If your total blood cholesterol exceeds 300 mg/dl, your risk of developing coronary heart disease is four times greater than that of someone whose cholesterol level is 200 mg/ dl.*

can take a blood sample from your finger or arm to determine your total cholesterol levels. Total blood cholesterol levels over 200 are now considered "borderline high," and levels exceeding 240 mg/dl are considered "high." Since blood cholesterol levels can vary (total cholesterol levels can vary by as much as 15 points in the same day), a second test may be needed to confirm elevated levels.

If your total blood cholesterol is more than 240 mg/dl or you have a family history of premature heart disease, your doctor may recommend that you undergo a *lipid profile,* a blood test in which the levels of several blood fats (*lipids*) are analyzed. This test gives more detailed information about your risk. Blood is drawn from a vein in your arm after you haven't eaten for at least 12 hours, and levels of very low density lipoproteins, low-density lipoproteins, high-density lipoproteins, and blood triglycerides are measured.

If you have either a family history of heart disease or high blood cholesterol levels, you may want to seek out a geneticist, a genetic counselor, and/or a physician who specializes in lipid disorders for further evaluation and treatment. (See Recommended Resources at the back of this book for help in finding these medical specialists.) *If someone in your family has a confirmed case of FH, all other immediate family members should be tested for the defect.*

CHOLESTEROL TESTS: WHAT THE
RESULTS MEAN

High total and LDL cholesterol levels raise your heart attack risk. However, the lower your HDL cholesterol level, the greater your risk of coronary heart disease.

You may notice that your LDL and HDL cholesterol values don't add up to your total blood cholesterol level. LDLs carry about 60 to 70 percent of the cholesterol, and HDLs carry about 25 percent; other lipoproteins carry the rest.

Total Cholesterol

below 200 mg/dl	desirable
200–240 mg/dl	borderline high
above 240 mg/dl	high

LDL Cholesterol

below 130 mg/dl	desirable
130–160 mg/dl	borderline high
above 160 mg/dl	high

HDL Cholesterol

below 35 mg/dl	increased risk
above 35 mg/dl	acceptable

OTHER RISK FACTORS FOR HEART DISEASE

Your family medical history and blood cholesterol levels are just two of many *risk factors* that can be used to determine your vulnerability to heart disease. You may have heard of many others, from coffee to allergies. Often, the studies reporting on these and other risk factors are still too preliminary for scientists to come to any firm conclusions. However, over the years, population studies have singled out a dozen or so risk factors that can be used to help predict the likelihood that someone will develop heart disease. These can be classified into two types: *major risk factors,* which are strongly associated with an increased risk of cardiovascular disease among large groups of people, and *contributing risk factors,* which also increase the risk of cardiovascular disease, but no one is sure of their precise role.

Some risk factors you can't do much about; others you can influence—and thereby significantly improve your odds against developing heart disease.

*   *   *

Major Risk Factors You Can't Change

Increasing age: Everybody's risk of heart disease increases with age. Nearly 55 percent of all heart attack victims are 65 or older; of those who die from heart attacks, about four out of five are over 65.

The increased risk with advancing age can be partly explained by the aging process itself. The connective tissues in the artery walls become stiffer with age, a condition known as "hardening of the arteries," or *arteriosclerosis*. As a result, blood pressure may rise, and the heart's workload may increase, causing the heart muscle to thicken and stiffen over time. As a general rule, blood pressure and blood cholesterol levels tend to rise with age, thus contributing to the increased risk.

Male sex: Although coronary heart disease is the leading cause of death and disability for both men and women, men are more vulnerable to heart disease than women. One in five men develops symptoms of heart disease before age 60, compared to one in 17 women. This means that men are two to three times more likely to develop heart disease than women. No one is sure exactly why women appear to be protected against heart disease, although researchers suspect that the reproductive hormone *estrogen* plays a role.

Major Risk Factors You Can Change

You can't change your genes, your age, or your gender, but you can influence the following risk factors:

High blood cholesterol: As you have already seen, your risk of heart disease increases along with rising blood cholesterol levels. And while it's true that your liver manufactures most of the cholesterol in your body, blood cholesterol levels are also affected by your diet and other outside influences.

The amount of fat and cholesterol in your diet—particularly saturated fats in meat and dairy products—plays a key role in elevating blood cholesterol levels. Cigarette smoking, exercise, and certain hormones affect blood cholesterol levels as well.

High blood pressure: Elevated blood pressure may be one of the most powerful contributors to cardiovascular disease. Even mild elevations in blood pressure lead to a greater incidence of premature atherosclerosis, heart attacks, and strokes. The greater the blood pressure, the greater the risk. And keeping blood pressure under control does lower the risk for both heart attacks and stroke.

Cigarette smoking: Although most people associate cigarette smoking with lung cancer, coronary heart disease is the largest smoking-related cause of death. Nearly three times more smokers die of heart disease than lung cancer. Your risk increases with the number of cigarettes you smoke. And when smoking is combined with other risk factors, your chances of developing heart disease skyrocket. Women who smoke and take birth control pills, which have also been associated with an increased risk of heart disease, are up to 39 times more likely to have a heart attack than women who don't. (More on the Pill later.) Cigarette smoking also increases the heart disease risk of nonsmoking family members who breathe secondhand smoke. Smokers who quit, however, cut their heart disease risk in half within two years.

Contributing Risk Factors

The connection between contributing risk factors and cardiovascular disease is not as well understood as that of the major risk factors listed above. Nevertheless, these conditions can substantially increase the chance that you'll develop heart disease, and treatment of them should be included in any program to reduce your risk.

Obesity: Being overweight (more than 30 percent over your "ideal" or "desirable" weight) increases your risk of heart disease even if you have no other risk factors. Excess weight increases the strain on the heart. Obesity also influences blood pressure and blood cholesterol and can lead to diabetes. Fat that accumulates around your waist appears to be more dangerous than fat that accumulates on the thighs and buttocks. Upper-body fat is associated with increased LDL cholesterol and lower HDL cholesterol and an increased risk of hypertension and diabetes.

Physical inactivity: Cholesterol gets all the attention these days, but a growing number of studies now show that sedentary living significantly raises your risk of developing coronary heart disease—perhaps even as much as high blood pressure, high blood cholesterol, and cigarette smoking.

Diabetes: More than 80 percent of people with diabetes die of some form of heart or blood vessel disease. One reason may be that diabetes affects cholesterol and triglyceride levels. Keeping diabetes in check helps reduce the risk, however.

Stress: Some scientists have noted a relationship between coronary heart disease risk and a person's life stress, personality traits, and socioeconomic status. Some people also respond to stress in negative ways—smoking and drinking more heavily than normal, for instance—and their *responses* to stress may ultimately be more risky than the stress itself.

It's hard to determine the extent to which stress influences the risk of heart disease, since most people respond to stress in different ways, and what's stressful to some may not be to others. But the evidence is convincing enough that you should not overlook stress as a possible risk factor.

CHILDREN AT RISK

Although heart disease usually doesn't strike until adulthood, the development of plaques on the artery walls may actually begin in childhood. This was one of the stunning findings to come out of a major ongoing study on heart disease and children in the town of Bogalusa, Louisiana. During the course of the study, thousands of black and white children—ranging in age from newborns through 26 years—were periodically screened for total and LDL cholesterol, blood pressure, and other risk factors for heart disease. The researchers also conducted autopsies on 44 youths who died in accidents or of illnesses other than cardiovascular disease and found that children as young as age 10 have fatty streaks in their arteries that are believed to later develop into artery-narrowing plaques.

The study came on the heels of a national campaign encouraging all Americans over 18 to "know your cholesterol number," and it raised many more questions than it answered: Should all children know their cholesterol number, too? Perhaps more important, would treating children with high cholesterol keep them from developing heart disease as adults?

Citing inaccuracies in the screening tests, the American Heart Association, the American Academy of Pediatrics, and other groups decided against screening all children for elevated blood cholesterol. However, the groups do advocate screening for some children. *You should notify your pediatrician if your child is over age two and his or her parents, grandparents, uncles, or aunts had or have*

- high cholesterol levels,
- early cardiovascular disease (under age 55 for men or under age 60 for women),
- a history of sudden heart attack or stroke, or
- other signs of atherosclerosis, such as angina.

Mass screening tests for cholesterol can sometimes be inaccurate, and children's cholesterol levels fluctuate quite a bit. (Diet, stress, exercise, puberty, and weight changes can influence a child's cholesterol levels.) At least one study suggests that some children with high cholesterol may outgrow the condition. For these reasons, children should undergo repeated measurements before a diagnosis is made. Youngsters with cholesterol levels above 170 mg/dl should also have their triglycerides and HDL cholesterol measured after an overnight fast. Even if total blood cholesterol measurements are normal, the American Heart Association and the American Academy of Pediatrics recommend remeasurements of "at risk" children every two to three years.

As with adults, high blood pressure, obesity, and cigarette smoking, in addition to high blood cholesterol, also put children and adolescents at greater risk. Children who have diabetes and children whose siblings have diabetes are also considered to have a higher risk of developing cardiovascular disease later in life.

As you'll see in the pages to come, treatment for children at risk is similar to that of adults—with a few important exceptions. Some studies have shown, for instance, that low-fat diets and other preventive measures that work well for adults may do more harm than good in some children, particularly those under age two. If your child has high blood cholesterol levels or other risk factors for heart disease, you *should not* attempt to treat it on your own. Plan to work closely with your pediatrician to manage your child's elevated risk factors.

RISKY BUSINESS

As you read through this chapter, you may have been tempted to do a little mental arithmetic to size up your risk of developing heart disease—and that of your family. However, gauging your risk isn't quite as simple as tallying up the various risk factors. To begin with, simply having one risk factor doesn't mean you'll automatically develop heart disease. Take high blood cholesterol, for instance. While it's indisputable that the risk of heart disease rises as blood cholesterol levels rise, *many people with high cholesterol do not develop heart disease, and many with low cholesterol levels do.* The point is that coronary heart disease is not a simple issue related only to blood cholesterol levels.

On the other hand, when two or more major risk factors are combined, the sum is often greater than the parts, and your odds of developing coronary heart disease jump even higher. For instance, with a high cholesterol level and high blood pressure, risk increases six-fold. If you also smoke, your risk increases more than 20-fold.

To get a rough idea of how at risk you are, complete the chart on the next few pages (called RISKO), a self-assessment test developed by the American Heart Association. Remember that RISKO will give you an estimate of your risk; it is not a substitute for a thorough physical examination and evaluation by your physician.

Now that you know where you and your family stand and which risk factors could stand improvements, let's look at some practical ways to start beating the odds.

RISKO

Men

Find the column for your age group. Everyone starts with a score of 10 points. Work down the page *adding* points to your score or *subtracting* points from your score.

1. Weight

Locate your weight category in the table on page 28. If you are in . . .

		54 or Younger	55 or Older
		Starting Score [10]	Starting Score [10]
☐	weight category A	Subtract 2	Subtract 2
☐	weight category B	Subtract 1	Add 0
☐	weight category C	Add 1	Add 1
☐	weight category D	Add 2	Add 3
		Equals ☐	**Equals** ☐

2. Systolic Blood Pressure

Use the "first" or "higher" number from your most recent blood pressure measurement. If you do not know your blood pressure, estimate it by using the letter for your weight category. If your blood pressure is . . .

		54 or Younger	55 or Older
A	119 or less	Subtract 1	Subtract 5
B	between 120 and 139	Add 0	Subtract 2
C	between 140 and 159	Add 0	Add 1
D	160 or greater	Add 1	Add 4
		Equals ☐	**Equals** ☐

3. Blood Cholesterol Level

Use the number from your most recent blood cholesterol test. If you do not know your blood cholesterol, estimate it by using the letter for your weight category. If your blood cholesterol is . . .

A	199 or less	Subtract 2	Subtract 1
B	between 200 and 224	Subtract 1	Subtract 1
C	between 225 and 249	Add 0	Add 0
D	250 or higher	Add 1	Add 0
		Equals ☐	**Equals** ☐

4. Cigarette Smoking

(If you smoke a pipe, but not cigarettes, use the same score adjustment as those cigarette smokers who smoke less than a pack a day.) If you . . .

☐	do not smoke	Subtract 1	Subtract 2
☐	smoke less than a pack a day	Add 0	Subtract 1
☐	smoke a pack a day	Add 1	Add 0
☐	smoke more than a pack a day	Add 2	Add 3
		Final Score Equals ☐	**Final Score Equals** ☐

Weight Table for Men

Look for your height (without shoes) in the far left column and then read across to find the category into which your weight (in indoor clothing) would fall.

Because both blood pressure and blood cholesterol are related to weight, an estimate of these risk factors for each weight category is printed at the bottom of the table.

Your Height FT IN		Weight Category (lbs) A	B	C	D
5	1	up to 123	124–148	149–173	174 plus
5	2	up to 126	127–152	153–178	179 plus
5	3	up to 129	130–156	157–182	183 plus
5	4	up to 132	133–160	161–186	187 plus
5	5	up to 135	136–163	164–190	191 plus
5	6	up to 139	140–168	169–196	197 plus
5	7	up to 144	145–174	175–203	204 plus
5	8	up to 148	149–179	180–209	210 plus
5	9	up to 152	153–184	185–214	215 plus
5	10	up to 157	158–190	191–221	222 plus
5	11	up to 161	162–194	195–227	228 plus
6	0	up to 165	166–199	200–232	233 plus
6	1	up to 170	171–205	206–239	240 plus
6	2	up to 175	176–211	212–246	247 plus
6	3	up to 180	181–217	218–253	254 plus
6	4	up to 185	186–223	224–260	261 plus
6	5	up to 190	191–229	230–267	268 plus
6	6	up to 195	196–235	236–274	275 plus
Estimate of Systolic Blood Pressure		119 or less	120 to 139	140 to 159	160 or more
Estimate of Blood Cholesterol		199 or less	200 to 224	225 to 249	250 or more

Women

Find the column for your age group. Everyone starts with a score of 10 points. Work down the page *adding* points to your score or *subtracting* points from your score.

1. Weight

Locate your weight category in the table on page 31. If you are in . . .

		54 or Younger	55 or Older
		Starting Score [10]	Starting Score [10]
[ ]	weight category A	Subtract 2	Subtract 2
[ ]	weight category B	Subtract 1	Subtract 1
[ ]	weight category C	Add 1	Add 1
[ ]	weight category D	Add 2	Add 1
		Equals [ ]	Equals [ ]

2. Systolic Blood Pressure

Use the "first" or "higher" number from your most recent blood pressure measurement. If you do not know your blood pressure, estimate it by using the letter for your weight category. If your blood pressure is . . .

		54 or Younger	55 or Older
A	119 or less	Subtract 2	Subtract 3
B	between 120 and 139	Subtract 1	Add 0
C	between 140 and 159	Add 0	Add 3
D	160 or greater	Add 1	Add 6
		Equals [ ]	Equals [ ]

3. Blood Cholesterol Level

Use the number from your most recent blood cholesterol test. If you do not know your blood cholesterol, estimate it by using the letter for your weight category. If your blood cholesterol is . . .

A	199 or less	Subtract 1	Subtract 3
B	between 200 and 224	Add 0	Subtract 1
C	between 225 and 249	Add 0	Add 1
D	250 or higher	Add 1	Add 3
		Equals ☐	**Equals** ☐

4. Cigarette Smoking

If you . . .

☐	do not smoke	Subtract 1	Subtract 2
☐	smoke less than a pack a day	Add 0	Subtract 1
☐	smoke a pack a day	Add 1	Add 1
☐	smoke more than a pack a day	Add 2	Add 4
		Final Score Equals ☐	**Final Score Equals** ☐

Weight Table for Women

Look for your height (without shoes) in the far left column and then read across to find the category into which your weight (in indoor clothing) would fall.

Because both blood pressure and blood cholesterol are related to weight, an estimate of these risk factors for each weight category is printed at the bottom of the table.

Your Height FT IN	Weight Category (lbs) A	B	C	D
4 8	up to 101	102–122	123–143	144 plus
4 9	up to 103	104–125	126–146	147 plus
4 10	up to 106	107–128	129–150	151 plus
4 11	up to 109	110–132	133–154	155 plus
5 0	up to 112	113–136	137–158	159 plus
5 1	up to 115	116–139	140–162	163 plus
5 2	up to 119	120–144	145–168	169 plus
5 3	up to 122	123–148	149–172	173 plus
5 4	up to 127	128–154	155–179	180 plus
5 5	up to 131	132–158	159–185	186 plus
5 6	up to 135	136–163	164–190	191 plus
5 7	up to 139	140–168	169–196	197 plus
5 8	up to 143	144–173	174–202	203 plus
5 9	up to 147	148–178	179–207	208 plus
5 10	up to 151	152–182	183–213	214 plus
5 11	up to 155	156–187	188–218	219 plus
6 0	up to 159	160–191	192–224	225 plus
6 1	up to 163	164–196	197–229	230 plus
Estimate of Systolic Blood Pressure	119 or less	120 to 139	140 to 159	160 or more
Estimate of Blood Cholesterol	199 or less	200 to 224	225 to 249	250 or more

WHAT YOUR SCORE MEANS

0-4   You have one of the lowest risks of heart disease for your age and sex.

5-9   You have a low to moderate risk of heart disease for your age and sex but there is some room for improvement.

10-14 You have a moderate to high risk of heart disease for your age and sex, with considerable room for improvement on some factors.

15-19 You have a high risk of developing heart disease for your age and sex with a great deal of room for improvement on all factors.

20 & over You have a very high risk of developing heart disease for your age and sex and should take immediate action on all risk factors.

Warning:

- If you have diabetes, gout, or a family history of heart disease, your actual risk will be greater than indicated by this appraisal.
- If you do not know your current blood pressure or blood cholesterol level, visit your physician or health center to have them measured. Then figure your score again for a more accurate determination of your risk.
- If you are overweight, have high blood pressure or high blood cholesterol, or smoke cigarettes, your long-term risk of heart disease is increased even if your risk in the next several years is low.

How to Reduce Your Risk

- Try to quit smoking permanently (see chapter 7).
- Have your blood pressure checked regularly, preferably every twelve months after age 40. If your blood pressure is high, see your physician. Remember blood pressure medicine is only effective if taken regularly.
- Consider your daily exercise (or lack of it). A half hour of brisk walking, swimming, or another activity should not be hard to fit into your day (see chapter 5).
- Give some serious thought to your diet. If you are over-

weight, or eat a lot of foods high in saturated fat or cholesterol (whole milk, cheese, eggs, butter, fatty foods, fried foods) then changes should be made in your diet (see chapter 3). Look for the *American Heart Association Cookbook* at your local bookstore.

- Visit or write your local Heart Association for further information and copies of free pamphlets on many related subjects including:
  - Reducing your risk of heart attack
  - Controlling high blood pressure
  - Eating to keep your heart healthy
  - How to stop smoking
  - Exercising for good health

Some Words of Caution

- If you have diabetes, gout, or a family history of heart disease, your real risk of developing heart disease will be greater than indicated by your RISKO score. If your score is high and you have one or more of these additional problems, you should give particular attention to reducing your risk.
- If you are a woman under 45 years or a man under 35 years of age, your RISKO score represents an upper limit on your real risk of developing heart disease. In this case, your real risk is probably lower than indicated by your score.
- Using your weight category to estimate your systolic blood pressure or your blood cholesterol level makes your RISKO score less accurate.
- Your score will tend to overestimate your risk if your actual values on these two important factors are average for someone of your height and weight.
- Your score will underestimate your risk if your actual blood pressure or cholesterol level is above average for someone of your height or weight.

CHAPTER
3

Diet: Your Primary Means of Prevention

I F you have high blood cholesterol, making a few changes in your diet may be all you need to do to lower your blood cholesterol to a safer level. In fact, people with the highest blood cholesterol levels often experience the greatest drop in blood cholesterol in response to dietary changes. And while a handful of people may see no change in blood cholesterol after changing their diet, over time, most people will experience an average reduction of 10 to 15 percent of total cholesterol—and lower levels of LDL cholesterol, too—by switching to a low-fat, low-cholesterol diet. This translates into a 20 to 30 percent reduction in heart disease risk, simply through diet therapy—one of the safest ways to prevent (and treat) hypertension, diabetes, and obesity, as well.

What's more, a "heart-healthy" diet—that is, a diet low in fat, cholesterol and sodium—can benefit the entire family, from ages two to 92. One of the most important contributions parents make to their children's health aside from their genes is a shared environment, of which diet is a major focus. Most health professionals now agree that, with caution, moderate cuts in fat probably won't harm most children—and may even help in a number of ways.

If the thought of changing what you eat makes you blanch, keep in mind that you won't necessarily be depriving yourself of food or flavor. On the contrary, as you can see from the following sample menus, *a low-fat diet actually allows you to eat more food.* That's because fat has more calories than protein or carbohydrate (there are nine calories in one gram of fat, compared with four in a gram of protein or carbohydrate). So when you take the fatty foods out of your diet, you can moderately increase the amount of low-fat foods you eat while still consuming the same amount of calories. (Of course, if you need to lose weight, you'll have to cut down on total calories as well, which we'll discuss further in chapter 5.)

As for flavor, there are now literally dozens of cookbooks (even a few gourmet cookbooks) featuring prudent and palatable low-fat, low-cholesterol dishes. (You'll find a few listed in the Recommended Resources at the back of the book.)

Less Fat, More Food

High-Fat Menu	Low-Fat Menu
Breakfast:	**Breakfast:**
1 fried egg	¾ cup cereal
2 slices bacon	⅓ cup strawberries
2 slices toast with 1 pat butter each	½ cup 1% milk
4 oz orange juice	½ bagel with jelly
black coffee	1 oz low-fat cream cheese
	4 oz orange juice
	black coffee
Mid-morning snack:	**Mid-morning snack:**
black coffee	6 oz low-fat fruited yogurt
1 jelly-filled doughnut	

Lunch:

1 3-oz hamburger
french fries
1 12-oz soft drink

Lunch:

3-oz water-packed tuna salad
    made with 1 tbs mayonnaise
    and 1 tbs low-fat yogurt on
    whole-wheat bread
carrot and celery sticks
1 apple
1 8-oz glass 1% milk

Dinner:

1 tossed salad with 2 tbs
    Thousand Island dressing
1 fried chicken breast
1 dinner roll
1 5-inch corn on the cob
1 tbs butter

Dinner:

½ cup cantaloupe
⅓ cup low-fat cottage cheese
1 skinless chicken breast sau-
    téed in olive oil and fresh
    herbs
1 cup spaghetti with tomato
    sauce and Parmesan cheese
½ cup steamed zucchini
1 Italian dinner roll
1 tbs butter (for bread, zuc-
    chini, and pasta)

Dessert:

½ cup vanilla ice cream

Dessert:

½ cup vanilla ice milk

2,000 calories
99 grams fat
44% calories from fat

2,000 calories
65 grams fat
29% calories from fat

CUTTING BACK ON DIETARY FAT

The most important dietary step you can take to protect
yourself from heart disease is to *cut down on the amount
of total and saturated fat in your diet.* Population studies
show that rates of coronary heart disease are relatively low
among cultures that consume low-fat diets. In Japan, where
coronary heart disease rarely develops, the average diet is
just 10 to 20 percent total fat and average blood cholesterol
levels are between 125 and 165 mg/dl. On the other hand,
the average American diet is about 38 percent fat, and average blood cholesterol levels are 205 mg/dl.

It's not just the total amount of fat you eat, but the kind of fat as well. All dietary fats consist of long chains of molecules known as fatty acids. There are three kinds of fatty acids, depending on the type and number of chemical "links" or bonds in the chain: *saturated, monounsaturated,* and *polyunsaturated.* Saturated fats, found mostly in meat and dairy products, raise your blood cholesterol more than anything else you eat. Apparently saturated fats decrease the number and/or the activity of LDL receptors in the liver. Dietary cholesterol in meat, dairy products, and eggs may elevate your blood cholesterol too.

On the other hand, polyunsaturated fats, the kind in most vegetable oils, have been found to lower blood cholesterol levels. Monounsaturated fats (such as olive and peanut oils), once thought to have no effect on blood cholesterol levels, are now believed to benefit the heart not only by lowering blood cholesterol but also by reducing blood pressure and blood sugar levels.

This is not to say, however, that you can eat large amounts of poly- and monounsaturated fats to bring your blood cholesterol levels down. Remember, the total amount of fat in your diet affects your blood cholesterol levels too. Most major health organizations advise that you limit the total amount of fat in your diet to no more than 30 percent of your daily calories. Saturated fats should be limited to less than 10 percent of total daily calories; polyunsaturated fats should be limited to 10 percent of calories as well. Mono-unsaturated fats should constitute between 10 and 15 percent of your total daily calories.

How to Get the Fat out of Your Diet

When cutting back on fat, by far the simplest way is to cut back on the foods that contribute the most total and saturated fat and cholesterol to your diet: meat, milk, and whole dairy products. That's not to say that you should *never* eat these foods. In fact, meat and dairy products are a valuable source of protein, vitamins, and minerals in your diet. Meat is high in iron and essential trace minerals. And milk and dairy products are some of the best food sources of calcium, needed for strong teeth and bones. Here are a few tips for striking a healthy balance with these foods:

Choose lean meats and the leanest cuts of meat: Poultry (with skin removed), fish, and veal are the leanest meats. Also look for lower grades of meat; choose "select" and "choice" grades over "prime" meats, which contain the most fat. Most shoppers usually purchase their meat by cut, not grade, however. When selecting cuts of meat, keep in mind the following guidelines:

- *Poultry.* Choose white meat over dark; a 3½-ounce roasted skinless chicken breast contains about half the fat of the same amount of dark meat (thigh and leg). The skin of chicken, turkey, and other types of poultry is high in fat, so *always* remove the skin before cooking.

- *Fish and shellfish.* Most fish is low in saturated fat and high in omega-3 fatty acids, a type of polyunsaturated fat that's believed to somehow protect against coronary artery disease. (We'll discuss fish oils in more detail later in this chapter.) Be aware that shrimp and squid are somewhat higher in cholesterol than other types of seafood, but they're still extremely low in fat.

- *Veal.* All trimmed cuts of veal (except chopped) are relatively low in fat.

- *Beef.* Round, sirloin, and loin are lowest in fat. Ground beef has the highest fat content. If you do use ground varieties of beef, choose ground round and ground sirloin. Try ground turkey, which has about one-fourth less fat (and costs less) than regular ground beef.

- *Pork.* Tenderloin and leg contain the least amount of fat, bacon and pork sausage the most.

- *Organ meats.* Liver, kidney, brain, tongue, and other organ meats are low in fat but high in cholesterol (one 3½-ounce serving of calf's liver contains 300 milligrams—the upper limit that most major health organizations recommend you eat in a day). So limit your consumption of these meats to about once a month.

- *Processed and luncheon meats.* Most are notoriously high in fat, not to mention sodium. One slice of beef bologna, for example, contains 6.5 grams of fat, meaning that 81 percent of its calories come from fat. (We will show you how to calculate "fat calories" later in this chapter.) Although several low-fat processed and luncheon meats are now available at the supermarket, be extra careful when choosing these products. Some luncheon meats, such as boiled ham, really are 98 percent fat free and may be a wise choice. However, some so-called "low-fat" chicken- and turkey-based cold cuts and franks contain just one or two grams less fat than all-beef versions, and the percentage of fat calories from these products is still high. For instance, a slice of turkey bologna contains 4.5 grams of fat—just 2 grams less than regular beef bologna—meaning that 67.5 percent of the calories still come from fat. As a rule, look for processed and luncheon meats containing no more than 3 grams of fat per ounce of meat. Best bets: boiled ham, honey loaf, and turkey breast.

Choose low-fat and no-fat milk and dairy products over whole dairy products: Skim milk contains no fat whatsoever and slightly more calcium than whole milk, making it the healthiest choice. Until you get used to the flavor of skim milk, use 1% milk. Don't be fooled by 2% fat milk. It doesn't have much less fat than whole milk, which contains 3.3% fat by volume.

When buying yogurt or cottage cheese, choose low-fat (1%

milk fat) or no-fat varieties as well. Few other cheeses are truly low in fat, so limit cheese in your diet, period.

When choosing ice cream or other frozen desserts, Popsicles, ice milk, low-fat frozen yogurt, sherbets, and sorbet are your lowest fat choices. A one-cup serving of vanilla ice milk contains just 5.6 grams of fat (27 percent of calories from fat), compared with a whopping 14.3 grams in a cup of regular vanilla ice cream (47 percent of calories from fat). Gourmet ice creams (such as Häagen-Dazs) contain the most fat, weighing in at a hefty 23.7 grams of fat per one-cup serving (61 percent of calories from fat).

Limit your consumption of egg yolks to two to three per week: One large egg contains 200 milligrams of cholesterol—two-thirds of the 300-milligrams-a-day limit. It's easy enough to find lower fat, lower cholesterol alternatives to the typical American bacon-and-eggs breakfast (see the preceding sample menu for a few suggestions). However, cutting back on the amount of eggs you use in cooking and baking may present a bigger challenge. Since virtually all of the cholesterol in eggs is in the yolk, one simple way to cut down on cholesterol in baked goods and egg dishes is to use egg whites instead of whole eggs. Two egg whites can be substituted for one whole egg in recipes. (Substituting two egg whites plus ½ to 1 teaspoon of oil works better in some recipes.)

Several brands of liquid, frozen, or powdered egg substitutes containing little or no cholesterol are available as well. Most are made from a base of egg whites and soy protein. Some contain vegetable oil, which adds a few more grams of fat and calories to the product.

Go vegetarian: Meat and dairy products may be good sources of protein, vitamins, calcium, and iron in your diet, but they're not the only ones. Many people find that avoiding meat (and sometimes dairy products) altogether is the easiest way to reduce the fat and cholesterol in their diets. If you're worried about getting enough protein in your diet by becoming a vegetarian, relax. Most Americans consume far more protein than they need. About 15 percent of the daily calories you consume should come from protein— which amounts to about 75 grams of protein on a 2,000-calorie-a-day diet, or two to three servings of high-protein foods daily. A one-cup serving of dried peas and beans (such as black beans, chickpeas, kidney beans, and lentils) contains as much protein as two ounces of meat—and virtually none of the fat or cholesterol. Tofu, a mild, cheese-like product made from the curds of soybean milk, is high in protein and calcium, and low in fat. Low-fat dairy products and eggs are also good sources of protein. (If you decide on the no-meat, no-dairy option, you should increase the number of protein servings to three or four per day.)

Keep in mind that protein from vegetables is "incomplete"—that is, it doesn't contain all of the nine essential amino acids your body needs from your diet to help build new tissue (or repair damaged tissue). Eating vegetable proteins together with other vegetables and/or whole grains (for instance, serving lentils over brown rice, or eating peanut butter on whole-grain bread) ensures that you're getting the full complement of amino acids.

Choose monounsaturated and polyunsaturated oils over margarine, and margarine over butter: Use polyunsaturated and monounsaturated oils instead of margarine or butter for baking and frying whenever possible. These include olive and peanut oils (monounsaturated) and safflower, sunflower, corn, and soybean oils (polyunsaturated).

For spreading, use margarine high in polyunsaturated fats instead of butter, which is high in both saturated fat and cholesterol. Choose liquid and tub margarine over stick forms. The softer or more fluid the margarine is, the less saturated it's likely to be. One recent study found that hardened vegetable oil containing *trans fatty acids* (formed when food companies add hydrogen to polyunsaturated and monounsaturated vegetable oils) raises LDL cholesterol levels and lowers HDL cholesterol when eaten in large amounts. Margarines made from safflower, sunflower, corn, and soybean oils are the lowest in saturated fat.

Sprinkle-on powders are ideal for seasoning hot, moist foods like baked potatoes and corn on the cob. However, the powders can't be used for frying or spreading. Check the label for the sodium content of powders as well.

Eat smaller portions of high-fat foods: This holds true especially for meat. Think of meat as a side dish rather than the main course of your meals. Two 3½-ounce portions of cooked meat or fish each day or one serving plus two 8-ounce glasses of milk will cover your daily need for protein. Smaller servings are considerably lower in fat and calories than the traditional 6- to 16-ounce slabs of meat you might be used to seeing on your plate. The right-sized serving of meat or fish will be about the size of a deck of playing cards or of the palm of your hand. Remember, too, that 4 ounces of lean boneless meat cooks down to about 3 ounces, as does 5 ounces of meat with bone.

Use reduced-fat cooking methods: Trim all visible fat from the meats you buy, and remove the skin from poultry before cooking. Broiling, roasting, stir frying, and stewing are best. When possible, cook meat on a rack so the fat drips down. Avoid panfrying or deep-frying.

You can also change recipes you know and love into low-fat, low-cholesterol recipes by using the following substitution guide:

When a recipe calls for . . .	Use . . .
1 tablespoon butter	1 tablespoon margarine or ¾ tablespoon oil*

1 cup shortening	⅔ cup vegetable oil
1 whole egg	2 egg whites
1 cup sour cream	1 cup yogurt (plus 1 table-spoon cornstarch for some recipes)
1 cup whole milk	1 cup 1% or skim milk

*Oil is best substituted only in recipes calling for melted butter.

Skip the cream sauces and creamy salad dressings: Top foods (fish and vegetables) with lemon juice and herbs instead of butter, sour cream, or heavy cream or cheese sauces. If you can't imagine eating a baked potato without butter, use a low-calorie margarine or sprinkle-on powder.

Watch out for hidden fat and cholesterol in baked goods: Commercially baked cakes, cookies, muffins, and breads are often made with saturated fat. Better to bake your own, using unsaturated oils and substituting egg whites for whole eggs (refer to the low-fat cooking guidelines just given).

Stay away from fast foods: Between 40 and 55 percent of the calories in most fast-food meals come from fat. Even such seemingly low-fat fare as chicken and fish contains quite a bit of fat. Chicken nuggets and chicken patty sandwiches often contain ground chicken skin. The total fat in six chicken nuggets is 20 grams, or 58 percent of the total calories. Fast-food establishments often fry their chicken and fish entrees in beef tallow, which adds saturated fat to the meal.

Many fast-food chains, bowing to criticisms about the questionable nutritional value of their foods, have begun to offer such low-fat alternatives as salads, low-fat dressings, fruit juice, and low-fat milk. These are excellent options when you find yourself in a fast-food restaurant. Look for fast-food restaurants that offer baked potatoes and/or salads, and choose one of these menu items instead of fries. Avoid topping your baked potato with butter, sour cream, cheese sauces, or chili. If you visit the salad bar, skip over such high-fat items as macaroni and potato salad and look for reduced-calorie salad dressings or oil and vinegar. If you order a sandwich, ask that it be made without added cheese or mayonnaise, which will reduce the fat content somewhat.

Counting Out Fat

If you require a more exact accounting of the fat in your diet, a convenient method is to count fat grams the same way you count calories on a weight-reducing diet. Most authorities recommend you limit fat to no more than 30 percent of your total daily calories. Thirty percent for someone who consumes about 1,500 calories a day is about 50 grams of fat. For every 100 calories above that, the daily fat allowance rises by about 3 grams.

Your age, body size, and activity level will determine the amount of calories you should consume each day. (A rough guide for people between the ages of 23 and 50 is to consume 2,000 to 2,700 calories per day.) Once you've determined your total daily calories, check the Fat Scorecard for the amount of fat you can eat (in grams) each day. Then simply keep track of your fat intake every day. You'll find the fat content of common foods in the Fat Finder's Guide in the Appendix at the back of the book. Many food labels now contain nutritional information, which lists the grams of fat per serving size.

Fat Scorecard

In a diet with daily calories of	Grams of fat that provide 30% of calories
1,500	50
2,000	67
2,500	83
3,000	100

HEAPING HELPINGS OF COMPLEX CARBOHYDRATES

If meat is a side dish, what's the main course? Complex carbohydrates, such as potatoes, rice, pasta, dried peas and beans, whole-grain breads, and fruits and vegetables. Not only are these foods naturally low in fat and calories, they're also high in vitamins and minerals and—perhaps more important—dietary fiber, a nutrient receiving increasing attention for its possible role in preventing heart disease.

Fiber is the indigestible part of fruits, vegetables, and grains. There are two types: *water-insoluble fiber* (found in whole grains, fruits, and vegetables) and *water-soluble fiber* (found in oats and oat bran, fruits, and dried peas and beans). Experts have long known that water-insoluble fiber helps relieve constipation, prevents hemorrhoids and diverticulosis (pouchlike sacs in the colon), and may also help prevent cancer of the colon. More recently, the focus has been on soluble fiber—*guar gum* (found in oat bran, rice bran, barley, and kidney beans), *psyllium seed* (found in Metamucil and other bulk fiber laxatives, as well as some breakfast cereals), and *pectin* (found in fruits)—and its potential for reducing blood cholesterol. Several studies have shown that when foods high in soluble fiber are added to a low-fat diet, they lower cholesterol levels of people with familial hypercholesterolemia by an average of 19 percent. And a study involving healthy people showed a more modest 3 percent decline in total cholesterol when 35 grams of oat bran were added to a low-fat diet. On the other hand, at least one recent study showed no difference whatsoever in the cholesterol-lowering ability of oat bran and a low-fiber wheat cereal, casting doubt on whether soluble fiber has any magical cholesterol-lowering properties.

Although several questions remain about the exact role of fiber in lowering cholesterol, complex carbohydrates are excellent substitutes for foods high in saturated fat and cholesterol. Foods of plant origin, like fruits, vegetables, grains, cereals, nuts, and seeds, contain no cholesterol. With a few exceptions (nuts and seeds, avocados and olives), these foods are very low in fat, too. And contrary to popular belief, high-carbohydrate foods such as pasta, rice, and potatoes are not fattening. These foods contain fewer calories than high-fat foods. What makes these foods fattening are the toppings we add: butter, cream sauces, whole milk or cream.

Try pasta, rice, and dried peas and beans (such as split peas, lentils, kidney beans, and navy beans) as main dishes, casseroles, soups, or other one-dish meals without high-fat sauces. Instead of having meat as a main course, use small quantities of meat, poultry, fish, or shellfish to add flavor to pasta and rice dishes and casseroles.

Except for granola, which often contains highly saturated coconut or coconut oil, most cereal products, both dry and cooked, are usually low in saturated fat and make a good stand-in for eggs at breakfast.

Breads and most rolls are low in fat. However, many other types of commercially baked goods are made with large amounts of saturated fat. Read the label to determine fat content. Stay away from croissants, biscuits, doughnuts, muffins, and butter rolls. By making your own baked goods, you can use unsaturated oils, skim milk, and egg whites.

Don't overdo it with fiber-rich foods, however. Most authorities recommend you limit your fiber intake to 20 to 30 grams a day (although they don't distinguish between soluble and insoluble fiber). Too much fiber in your diet can cause you to excrete other nutrients, notably calcium.

*   *   *

THE SODIUM CONNECTION

You have undoubtedly heard by now that a diet high in sodium (a main ingredient of table salt) raises your risk of high blood pressure. We now know that this is true only in a susceptible minority of people who are genetically salt-sensitive. For these people, cutting down on sodium can make a real difference, lowering blood pressure significantly and often reducing the need for antihypertensive medication.

Since we don't have any way of identifying who these "sodium-sensitive" people are, however, it makes sense to limit the amount of sodium in your diet. Most of us consume between 3,000 and 6,000 milligrams of sodium a day. Yet the National Research Council estimates that we need only 500 to 2,400 milligrams.

Foods highest in sodium are processed, prepackaged, and fast foods, which, as you've already seen, are high in fat as well. By cooking foods yourself and cutting down on the amount of salt used in cooking, you'll automatically reduce your sodium intake. Use plenty of herbs and spices when cooking, and look for no-sodium food seasonings in the store. By seasoning your food at the table with the salt shaker rather than adding salt to recipes when cooking, you'll use considerably less salt as well.

A FEW WORDS ABOUT OAT BRAN, FISH OILS, COFFEE, AND CHOLESTEROL

In recent years, there has been no shortage of reports on the effects of various foods on your heart: Oat bran lowers cholesterol. Fish oils are good for your heart. The headlines about coffee's role in heart disease seem to change every day. Indeed, over the last 10 years, it has become increasingly difficult to separate fact from fiction (and sometimes downright fraud) about health claims associated with the foods we eat.

Most of these claims contain a germ of truth. Unfortunately, however, the media tends to gloss over some of the facts. And food manufacturers, intent on cashing in on health-conscious consumers, have taken full advantage of consumer confusion and lax government regulations regarding food labeling. As a result, a number of food fads have come into vogue. Before you buy into the headlines and hype, make sure you've got all the facts about these fads:

Oat bran: When the National Heart, Lung, and Blood Institute announced in 1987 that just about half of all Americans needed to lower their cholesterol to reduce their risk of heart disease, the stage was set for one of the hottest-selling food items since sliced bread—oat bran. Seemingly overnight, new oat bran products began appearing on supermarket shelves, even though some important questions remained unanswered about the role of oat bran in lowering cholesterol. For instance, one study found essentially the same drop in blood cholesterol—about 7 percent—regardless of whether the volunteers ate a diet supplemented with oat bran or with low-fiber refined wheat products.

Also, no one knows yet how much oat bran is needed to achieve the cholesterol-lowering effect. Study participants with familial hypercholesterolemia ate a whopping 100 grams of oat bran a day—equivalent to a one-ounce bowl of pure oat bran cereal and five oat bran muffins—to lower their cholesterol by 19 percent. To add to the confusion, in one highly publicized study, a bowl of oatmeal containing just 9 grams of oat bran appeared to be as effective at lowering blood cholesterol as a bowl of oat bran cereal containing 28 grams of pure oat bran. Keep in mind that there's something food manufacturers won't tell you about their oat bran products: many food items—particularly oat bran muffins, cookies, snack crackers, and chips—contain enough fat to cancel out any potential cholesterol-lowering benefits that oat bran may have. Check the label for fat content before you buy.

Remember, too, that if future research shows that soluble fiber *is* responsible for lowering blood cholesterol, several foods besides oat bran are also high in soluble fiber. Dried peas and beans—including black and kidney beans, split peas, lentils, and chickpeas—contain the soluble fiber *beta glucan*. Rice bran and psyllium seed, now finding their way into some breakfast cereals, are also high in soluble fiber. Until we know more, it doesn't hurt to eat foods high in soluble fiber, since they're also naturally low in fat. But don't feel obligated to load up on oat bran products, which generally cost more than foods in which oat bran hasn't been added. Instead, eat a variety of foods high in both soluble and insoluble fiber, including plenty of dried peas and beans.

Fish oils: The fish oil fad began innocently enough. Researchers reported that heart attacks were almost unheard of among Greenland Eskimos, whose diet was made up almost exclusively of high-fat, high-cholesterol whale and seal meat and fish. Another study by researchers in Denmark suggested that the key to the Eskimos' healthy hearts might be a class of polyunsaturated fats known as omega-3 fatty acids. Apparently, if you eat enough of them, omega-3 fatty acids (*eicosapentaenoic acid,* or EPA, and *docosahexaenoic acid,* or DHA) lower cholesterol just like the polyunsaturated fats in vegetable oils.

Based on these and other preliminary reports about the heart-healthy benefits of fish oils, the market for fish oil supplements skyrocketed. By 1987, sales of fish oil capsules had reached $45 million. Many manufacturers claimed, among other things, that the supplements could lower cholesterol. However, in 1988, the U.S. Food and Drug Administration began cracking down on the makers of fish oil supplements, saying there wasn't enough strong evidence to support the health claims being made about the products. Moreover, no one knew the long-term effects of taking the supplements.

We now know that in small doses (10 capsules a day— the recommended amount) fish oil capsules *don't* lower blood cholesterol. However, omega-3 fatty acids may protect against heart disease in other ways. For instance, fish oils lower triglycerides in people whose levels are high to begin with. Twenty capsules a day (about two times the recommended dose) appear to lower blood pressure in some people. Animal studies suggest that fish oils may somehow prevent the buildup of plaque on the artery walls, possibly by making blood platelets (which control blood clotting) less sticky. Some evidence that fish oils exert an effect on the arteries themselves comes from studies involving patients who undergo *balloon angioplasty* (in which a balloon is inserted into a coronary artery and inflated to unblock the artery). In one study, those who took fish oil supplements were less likely to have the arteries close up again after the procedure, which normally occurs 25 to 40 percent of the time.

Should you take fish oil supplements? Most experts are hesitant to say yes, since so many of the studies are preliminary. And the supplements have side effects as well, including loose stools, belching, abdominal distension, and a possible increased need for vitamin E. Supplements containing cod liver oil also contain high amounts of vitamins A and D, which can be toxic at doses of 20 capsules a day. Until we know more, stick with fish—two to three times a week.

Coffee: So many conflicting reports have come out on the effects of coffee on heart disease risk that they've probably left you totally bewildered.

Why all the confusion? To begin with, coffee contains some 500 different chemicals, including caffeine. Many of the earlier studies didn't take into account the fact that there are several kinds of coffee beans and numerous ways of brewing coffee. For instance, about 85 percent of American coffee drinkers use the drip method, in which hot water passes through the coffee grounds one time. Scandinavians, on the other hand, usually boil either whole or coarsely ground beans in water, producing a much different and stronger brew. In fact, the differences in brewing methods probably account for the findings in one Scandinavian study, which showed increased blood cholesterol levels among drinkers of regular boiled coffee.

However, one of the largest and best-designed studies to date conducted by researchers at the Harvard University School of Public Health has cleared regular caffeinated coffee of causing heart troubles. According to this study, three or four cups a day of typical American coffee are safe for virtually everybody, even people with heart disease.

Decaffeinated coffee is another story. Both the Harvard study and another study from Stanford University found an increased risk of heart disease among heavy drinkers of decaffeinated coffee. The Harvard study showed that drinking four or more cups of decaffeinated coffee was associated with a moderate elevation in the risk of coronary heart disease and total cardiovascular disease (including stroke). The Stanford researchers reported that decaffeinated coffee raised levels of LDL cholesterol by an average of 9 mg/dl.

The researchers cautioned, however, that the statistical link between decaffeinated coffee and heart disease is weak, and more research is needed before firm conclusions can be made. For now, it seems that moderate amounts of regular drip-method coffee are safe, and there appears to be no particular reason to switch from regular to decaffeinated coffee to prevent heart disease.

*   *   *

READING BETWEEN THE LINES OF FOOD LABELS

Almost as confusing as food fads are food labels and the health claims made on them. In an effort to crack down on misleading food labels, the U.S. Food and Drug Administration has proposed 21 new regulations that would, among other things, require that nutrition labels appear on virtually all processed foods. (This is now done only on a voluntary basis.) The proposed regulations would also define ambiguous terms used on food labels, such as "free" (as in "cholesterol free") "low" (as in "low-fat") or "light." However, the new regulations probably won't be made final until late 1992, and may not go into effect until June 1993. So the confusion continues. For instance, as the regulations stand now, products claiming to have "no cholesterol" or "low cholesterol" may still be high in fat, including saturated fat. If there's a nutrition label, check the amount of fat in the product. If not, you'll have to rely on the ingredients list.

Unfortunately, while all products containing fat must specify the type of fat used in the ingredients list, the labels don't have to divulge the amount of fat in the product. As a rule, avoid or use sparingly products that list the following on ingredient labels:

- Animal fats (such as bacon fat, beef fat, chicken fat, lard, or suet),
- Butter,
- Coconut or coconut oil,
- Cream and cream sauce,
- Egg and egg yolk solids,
- Hydrogenated (hardened) fats or oils,
- Malted milk, milk chocolate, or cocoa butter,
- Palm or palm kernel oil, and
- Powdered whole-milk solids.

Instead, look for products that don't contain fat, or those that list only partially hydrogenated vegetable oils (cottonseed and/or soybean oil).

If a product does contain a nutrition label, it will probably list only the grams of fat found in the product, which is better than nothing, but still doesn't tell you much. To see whether the product is high in fat, you'll have to calculate the percentage of calories in the food that comes from fat, or the *fat calories*. The formula is simple: Multiply the grams of fat per serving by 9 (the number of calories in one gram of fat). Then divide that number by the total number of calories in a serving, and multiply by 100.

Here's an example, using a serving of canned beef ravioli in tomato sauce containing 6 grams of fat and 180 calories per serving:

$$
\begin{aligned}
& 6 \text{ (grams of fat per serving)} \\
\times\ & 9 \text{ (calories in 1 gram of fat)} \\
=\ & 54 \text{ (fat calories)} \\
\div\ & 180 \text{ (total calories)} \\
=\ & .30 \\
\times\ & 100 \\
=\ & 30 \text{ (percentage of calories from fat)}
\end{aligned}
$$

A PRUDENT DIET FOR CHILDREN

If your child has been found to have high blood cholesterol, it's best to work closely with your pediatrician—and perhaps even consult a pediatric dietitian—to develop a sensible low-fat eating plan that can be followed without too many tears. As we pointed out earlier, cutting too many calories and too much fat from a child's diet can do more harm than good, especially among underweight children or those under age two. Your pediatrician or a registered dietitian specializing in children's nutrition will be able to help you determine what dietary measures you need to take to help bring your child's cholesterol down.

On the other hand, most authorities now agree that *modest* reductions in fat are safe for almost all children over age two—even those who don't have high blood cholesterol levels. And there are plenty of compelling reasons to start good eating habits early. Researchers believe that elevated blood cholesterol levels in the majority of adults are largely a result of eating habits developed from birth. And as you may recall, fatty streaks in the coronary arteries that eventually lead to atherosclerosis have been seen in children as young as age 10.

Dietary guidelines for children over age two are essentially the same as they are for adults: No more than 30 percent of total calories should come from fat, and no more than 10 percent of fat calories should come from saturated fat. Cholesterol should be limited to 100 milligrams per 1,000 calories daily, not to exceed 300 milligrams a day. Most of the same recommendations for adults apply to kids, too: Substitute red meat with chicken, turkey, or fish; switch to lower fat milk; bake with unsaturated oils; buy goods that have been prepared with vegetable oils (and not coconut or palm oil).

MAKING LASTING CHANGES

Changing your eating habits may seem like a monumental task, especially when your goal is to make the changes last for the rest of your life. Be patient with yourself. Remember, while eating some foods high in saturated fat and cholesterol for one day or at one meal won't raise your blood cholesterol levels, resuming your old eating habits will. Plus, as you gradually adapt to the new low-fat foods, you may be pleasantly surprised to find your food preferences have changed. You may no longer think of your new way of eating as a diet but part of your regular routine. Here are a few tips for making the changes last a lifetime.

- Set goals for cholesterol levels and weight. Before you start your cholesterol-lowering diet, your physician will measure your cholesterol levels and help you set a goal for the total and LDL cholesterol levels that are right for you. Your doctor will also help you choose a sensible time frame to work within. If weight is a problem, your doctor can help you target an appropriate goal for weight loss as well. (We'll discuss weight-loss methods in chapter 5.)

- Make changes gradually. You'll be more likely to stick with your new low-fat diet if you slowly adapt to new eating habits over time. For instance, if you're in the habit of drinking whole milk, ease your way to skim milk by switching to 2% milk for a few weeks, then 1% milk, and finally skim milk.

- Monitor your progress. Have your cholesterol level checked periodically by your doctor—every three to six months if your blood cholesterol is particularly high.

- Don't be discouraged if you're not an "overnight success." It takes time to make dietary changes, and even more time to see the results of those changes. Some people won't see a significant change in their blood cholesterol levels for up to a year after instituting dietary measures. Others may find they have to cut even more than 30 percent of the fat from their diets before blood cholesterol levels go down. Still others find that working with a qualified dietitian gets results—even after their own efforts have failed. (To find a qualified dietitian, check the Recommended Resources at the back of this book.) The bottom line is that most people *will* eventually experience a drop in their blood cholesterol levels and their risk of heart disease by switching to a low-fat diet. You can too.

CHAPTER

4

The Fitness Factor

ANY sensible program for managing your risk of heart disease should factor in plenty of physical activity. Scientists at the Centers for Disease Control in Atlanta, reviewing some 43 population studies, found that *sedentary people were nearly twice as likely to develop coronary heart disease as those who regularly exercised for at least 20 minutes three times a week.* The CDC review included one landmark study by Harvard University's Dr. Ralph Paffenbarger, who showed that the risk of heart attack was reduced by as much as 50 percent in more active men compared with sedentary men. Dr. Paffenbarger found that even leisure-time activities, such as gardening, bowling, and bicycling were associated with a decreased risk.

Exercise appears to guard against heart disease in several ways:

- Regular physical activity raises levels of HDL cholesterol, the "good" cholesterol believed to protect against heart disease. Active people have higher levels of HDL cholesterol than inactive people. When sedentary people begin to exercise, their HDL cholesterol rises an average five to six points over the course of a year.

- A regular program of aerobic exercise lowers your blood pressure and heart rate, allowing the heart to pump blood more efficiently.

- Exercise burns body fat, which helps counter the secondary risk factor of obesity.

- Your body uses insulin more efficiently when you exercise, which may lower your risk of developing non-insulin dependent diabetes.

You don't need to become a marathon runner to reap the benefits of exercise on your heart and health. In fact, as you'll soon discover, a sedentary life-style may be one of the easiest risk factors to change.

HOW MUCH IS ENOUGH?

Although any kind of physical activity is better than none, some activities are clearly better than others. Most doctors recommend aerobic activities—those that involve increasing your heart rate and breathing and using the large muscles of your body—for the most protection. Brisk walking, jogging or running, bicycling, swimming, and aerobic dancing are considered aerobic activities. Nonaerobic activities, such as weight lifting and stretching exercises, may increase your muscle strength and flexibility, but they do little to increase the efficiency of the most important muscle in your body: your heart.

It's not just the type of activity you engage in that confers protection against heart disease but also how strenuously you exercise and how often. You'll need to raise your heart rate to a working level—typically 60 to 80 percent of its maximum capacity—to give your heart and lungs a sufficient workout. And you'll need to sustain the activity for at least 15 to 20 minutes each time. For optimal results, you should plan on exercising at this level at least three times a week.

BEFORE YOU BEGIN

Before you embark on an exercise program, a consultation with your doctor is recommended—especially if you've got an elevated risk of heart disease and have been sedentary for more than a year. The reason: some often symptomless physical conditions may make exercise too dangerous for you. Other conditions may limit the amount of exercise you can do or may require that you exercise only under a doctor's care. For instance, while exercise is a great way to help control mildly to moderately high blood pressure, you should do so only under a doctor's supervision. If you have severely high blood pressure (200/100), however, you should not exercise at all, since exercise itself temporarily elevates blood pressure and could trigger a heart attack or stroke. Likewise, if you have angina or another heart condition, *thrombophlebitis* (blood clots in the legs), uncontrolled diabetes, or musculoskeletal problems that interfere with exercise, you may be advised not to exercise.

If you have a family history of heart disease, your doctor may recommend that you undergo an electrocardiogram (ECG), an exercise stress test, and tests for blood cholesterol, triglycerides, and blood glucose (blood sugar) levels, if you haven't had them already. If you already have coronary artery disease, you'll probably undergo these tests, as well as a chest X ray and possibly a cardiac echogram.

DO YOU NEED AN EXERCISE STRESS TEST?

If you're over 35 and have one or more risk factors for heart disease (family history, elevated cholesterol levels, obesity, smoking, or high blood pressure), you should undergo an exercise stress test before starting an exercise program. This test is essentially an electrocardiogram that measures your heart rate and electrical activity while you work out on a treadmill or stationary bicycle. The test can detect problems that a "resting" ECG can't. For example, your heart may be receiving sufficient oxygen while you're at rest; however, when you begin exercising, the ECG may show that your heart isn't getting enough oxygen. Typically this is caused by the narrowing of arteries as a result of plaque buildup on the artery walls.

The test is also used as a screening device for people about to begin an exercise program. Even if you're found to have evidence of heart disease, the test results can be used to tailor an exercise program to your individual needs.

The American College of Sports Medicine also recommends that you have an exercise stress test if you're over 45—regardless of whether you have any known risk factors for heart disease or whether you've been regularly exercising for years. The test is even more important if you're over 45 and don't exercise but would like to begin. On the other hand, there's no scientific evidence that the test benefits anyone under age 35, even if they have risk factors for heart disease.

The test itself is fairly straightforward. Before the test begins, a number of sensors or "leads" are placed on your chest to transmit signals to a machine that records your heart's activity on graph paper. Then you'll begin exercising on an automated treadmill or stationary bicycle, which will gradually speed up your pace. The ECG monitors your heart's rhythm and its electrical activity; your pulse and blood pressure will be monitored too. Generally, you exercise for about 10 or 15 minutes, or until fatigue keeps you from continuing or warning symptoms appear (shortness of breath, dizziness, chest pains, abnormal blood pressure or heart rate or rhythm, nausea).

Exercise tests aren't perfect. A number of studies have reported high false-positive results—in other words, the test indicates signs of heart disease in healthy people. The test may also fail to detect some cases of heart disease. In spite of these flaws, the exercise stress test remains a worthwhile screening device, and can be particularly helpful in determining how strenuously and for how long beginners should exercise.

MAKING A TIME COMMITMENT

Your first priority in launching an exercise program will be to make a time commitment. As we pointed out earlier in this chapter, 20 minutes of aerobic activity three times a week is a good goal. Your program should also include a 10-minute warm-up and a 10- to 15-minute cool-down period, meaning that you should allow roughly 40 to 50 minutes for each exercise session.

Most people can't seem to find the time to exercise, but if you have an increased risk of heart disease, you may simply have to make time. Get up a half-hour earlier and exercise in the morning before going to work. Or take a brisk 45-minute walk on your lunch hour.

FINDING YOUR TARGET HEART RANGE

You'll need to know your target heart rate before you begin exercising to ensure that you're getting a proper workout. For most healthy people this means exercising strenuously enough to raise your heart rate to 60 to 80 percent of its maximum capacity. If you don't exercise within your target range, the amount of cardiovascular conditioning—and protection from heart disease—may be negligible. On the other hand, too strenuous a workout can put too much strain on your heart.

Your target heart rate is actually not a single number but a range between two numbers, which you should aim for when exercising. If you have an exercise stress test, your physician can use the results to help determine your target range. If you don't have an exercise test, use the formula here to calculate your target range.

220 − your age × (.60 to .80) = your target heart range

Here's an example for a 40-year-old man or woman:

$$220 - 40 = 180 \times (.60 \text{ to } .80) = 108 \text{ to } 144.$$

This person's target heart range is between 108 and 144 pulse beats per minute.

You can measure your heart rate while exercising by taking your pulse at either the *carotid artery* in your neck or the *radial artery* in your wrist (fig. 4). To measure your carotid pulse, place the first two fingers (not the thumb) of your right hand on the left side of your throat; for the radial pulse, place the same two fingers on your left wrist on the thumb side. Using a digital watch that shows seconds, or a clock with a second hand, count your pulse for 10 seconds, then multiply the number of pulse beats you counted by six. Your pulse beats should fall somewhere within your target heart range.

CHOOSING AN ACTIVITY

When developing an exercise program, choose an activity that you enjoy doing. Here are some pros and cons of the most popular types of aerobic exercises.

Walking: This activity is the easiest and most convenient because you can walk practically anywhere, and walking requires no special skills or equipment; just comfortable, loose-fitting clothes and a good pair of walking shoes (wear

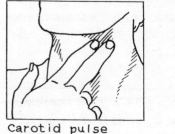 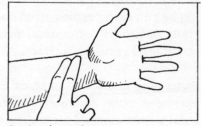

Carotid pulse   Radial pulse

FIGURE 4. How to Take Your Pulse.

shoes with a flexible, cushioned sole). Walking is less likely to cause injury as well, since it's a low-impact activity that doesn't put too much strain on your muscles and joints. Your biggest concern will be ensuring that you walk briskly enough to get a cardiovascular workout. Monitor your heart rate while you walk and pick up the pace if your heart rate doesn't reach its working range after 10 minutes or so. For a more intensive workout, swing your arms as you walk, plan your walk along a hilly route, or wear specially designed wrist and/or ankle weights. (Note, though, that the added weight of wrist and ankle weights may increase your risk of injury.)

Jogging and running: An excellent way to get a good aerobic workout, jogging and running also carry a much greater risk of injury than walking, particularly muscle strains, knee injuries, and stress fractures of the lower legs and feet. These activities also require special footwear designed to help absorb some of the shock of this high-impact activity. Look for running shoes with a wide base for stability, a cushioned sole for shock absorption, and plenty of flexibility.

When jogging or running, proper form is important too. Hold your body erect, keeping your arms, shoulders, and neck relaxed. Your arms should swing directly forward and backward, not across your body. Keep your elbows slightly flexed, and don't clench your fists. To track your progress, jog or run on a premeasured course—either a track or specially designed par-course, preferably with an even, relatively level running surface.

Swimming and water aerobics: Swimming and other aquatic exercises, such as water dancing, give a good cardiovascular workout while protecting your joints from the jarring movements of other aerobic activities. And these activities give your whole body a workout.

You don't necessarily have to know how to swim in order to work out in the water. Many fitness clubs, municipal pools, the YMCA and YWCA now offer water aerobics classes in which you hold onto the side of the pool or stand in shallow water (up to your shoulders) as you perform leg lifts and other aerobic and/or dance routines.

The biggest drawback to water-based activities may be having year-round access to a swimming pool or other body of water (such as a lake or ocean) in which to perform them. Again, check with local fitness clubs or your local YMCA or YWCA to see if an indoor pool is available for use during inclement weather.

Bicycling: If you have a bicycle in good working condition, cycling can be a simple and enjoyable way to work out. Like walking, bicycling doesn't put too much strain on your joints. To ensure you're getting a good workout, keep track of the amount of time you spend cycling and monitor your heart rate to make sure it reaches its target range. If your heart rate is too low, pedal harder (or switch to a higher gear).

A stationary bicycle allows you to exercise even in poor weather and/or after dark, when cycling outside can be hazardous. Set up a television set near the bike and watch the evening news while you work out!

Aerobic dance: Fitness clubs and municipal recreation centers usually offer a wide variety of aerobics classes to suit your fitness level and time schedule. Low-impact aerobics is somewhat kinder to your joints, requiring that you keep one foot on the floor at all times. High-impact aerobics involves more jarring movements, such as jumping, kicking, and jogging. The risk of injury is high in aerobics classes, particularly high-impact classes. To minimize your risk:

- Make sure your instructor is trained and qualified to lead classes. Look for instructors who have been certified by the American College of Sports Medicine, the Aerobic Fitness Association of America, or the International Dance Education Association.

- Check out the room in which the classes will be held as well. The best surface is a suspended wood floor; the worst is concrete.

WARMING UP AND COOLING DOWN

Your exercise routine should include a warm-up and cooldown period preceding and following your aerobic workout. A 5- to 10-minute warm-up of stretching exercises and moderate aerobic activity increases the blood flow to your heart and muscles and lessens the shock of sudden strenuous activity to your heart. Warming up before strenuous activity also increases the flexibility of your muscles and joints, which may help reduce your risk of injury.

A 5- to 10-minute cool-down period after an aerobic workout is essential too. If you stop cold, the extra blood diverted to your muscles during exercise may pool in your legs, causing a dangerous shortage of blood to either the brain or your heart. Decreased blood flow to the brain may cause you to feel dizzy or even pass out. Insufficient blood flow to the heart could lead to dangerous *arrhythmias* (irregular heartbeats). The cool-down period also helps your body cool off and helps stave off the buildup of lactic acid in the muscles, a major cause of post-exercise muscle soreness. Walking is an ideal way to cool down. Whatever you do, keep moving until your heart rate comes down below your target range.

GETTING STARTED

The watchword for beginning an exercise program is "go slowly." By starting out slowly, you give your body a chance to adjust to your new level of activity. You'll also be less likely to suffer from sore muscles—a major hurdle that stops many would-be exercisers from continuing beyond the first week of an exercise program. Perhaps more important, you'll decrease your risk of suffering an exercise-related injury, which could put you out of commission for weeks.

If you've been sedentary for more than a year but are otherwise healthy, try exercising for brief periods of time— say 10 to 15 minutes of aerobic activity, plus warm-up and cool-down—five or six times a week. You can gradually build up the amount of aerobic activity you do as you become more physically fit. This way, even if you miss a day or two, you'll still be exercising the minimum three days a week needed to keep your heart healthy.

KEEPING YOUR INTEREST HIGH

Aerobic exercises are repetitious by nature and can become monotonous. To ensure long-term success, try these tips:

- *Set realistic goals.* Your goals should match your abilities—don't set your sights on running three miles a day during the first week of your exercise program if you haven't been physically active in years. You're bound to be disappointed and discouraged from continuing your exercise program. (Most experts recommend that beginners literally walk for several weeks before they run.) Your doctor can help you determine what's realistic for you. Once you've reached these goals, work up some more.

- *Monitor your progress.* Keep track of your activities using the exercise diary on page 66. This will help reinforce your new habit by allowing you to see how your fitness level is improving each week. After every exercise session, record the date of your session, your activity, your exercise heart rate, how long and/or how far you performed your activity, and any comments you have about the session. For instance, you may want to record

Physical Activity Progress Report

Weekly goal _____

Day Date	Activity	Heart Rate	Distance Duration	Comments

the number of calories you burned (you'll find a calorie expenditure chart in the Appendix), whether you felt tired during the exercise session, how long it's been since you last exercised, and so on.

- *Choose an activity you enjoy and one that's convenient for you.* If you love to swim but don't have ready access to a swimming pool, chances are you won't swim as regularly as you should to keep your heart healthy. Choose another activity as a "backup" for the days you can't go swimming.

- *Vary your routine.* To keep from getting bored, alter your route or your routine from time to time. Or try varying your activities—if you're tired of walking, ride your bicycle instead.

- *Exercise with a partner.* This way, if your enthusiasm wanes, your partner may provide the incentive you need to go on, and vice versa. Make sure you and your partner are well matched in terms of fitness level and abilities, however. It can be discouraging to try to keep up with a marathon runner when you're more suited for a slow walk/jog around the block.

- *Reward yourself.* After you've faithfully followed your exercise routine for a month or two, treat yourself to a new outfit, a movie, or some other reward. Do the same after six months, and again after a year.

FROM INACTIVITY TO ACTIVITY

If you simply can't fit a regular exercise routine into your life, you can still become more physically active. Instead of hiring the boy next door to cut your grass, mow the lawn yourself. Take the stairs instead of the elevator at work. Leave your car at home and walk or ride your bicycle to the store. As we pointed out earlier, any activity is better than none.

CHAPTER
5

Reducing Your Weight and Your Odds

IF you're more than 30 percent over your ideal weight for your height, getting your weight under control should be a top priority. Overweight people are two to three times more likely to have high blood cholesterol levels, and three times more likely to develop high blood pressure and diabetes, than normal weight people. And remember that being overweight in itself may increase your risk of heart disease by putting more strain on your heart and arteries.

Upper-body weight—fat that accumulates around your waist—appears to be more hazardous to your health than fat that accumulates on the thighs and buttocks. Studies have associated upper-body fat with increased LDL cholesterol, decreased HDL cholesterol, and an increased risk of hypertension and diabetes.

Losing weight in itself is often enough to lower elevated blood cholesterol and blood pressure, and to keep non-insulin dependent diabetes in check without drugs and their sometimes serious side effects. One recent Harvard University study estimated that *as much as 70 percent of coronary disease in the obese could be prevented through weight loss alone.*

Don't be too discouraged by new findings that obesity is

hereditary. Again, most studies suggest that many over-weight people have a genetic predisposition to obesity that can be influenced by the environment. And while it's true that some people will lose weight more readily than others, most people will see some improvement in their weight by making a concerted effort. If you don't reach your ideal weight, remember that even a small drop in your weight will help lower blood cholesterol and blood pressure levels and help protect against the onset of diabetes.

ADOPTING A SENSIBLE STRATEGY

Theories abound about why people become obese. Not long ago, the prevailing wisdom was that overweight people suffered from deep-seated emotional problems that caused them to eat more food. We now know that obesity is a much more complex problem, involving a combination of genetic, metabolic, environmental, psychological, and sociological factors.

The confusion about just what causes obesity has also given rise to an equally confusing number of diet strategies—most of which don't work and some of which may be downright dangerous. Fasting has been abandoned by nearly all professionals as most of the weight lost during the first two weeks of a fast is water, which results in dangerous disturbances in electrolyte balance. Very low calorie diets (800 calories a day or less) are recommended only for very obese people whose other dieting efforts have failed. Such diets should be undertaken only under a doctor's supervision. "High-protein" diets are nutritionally inadequate and may lead to *ketosis,* an abnormal accumulation of chemicals called ketones in the body, which could lead to coma and even death.

With all the contradictory research and advice about obesity, one fact remains clear: excess body fat almost always results from chronically taking in more calories through food than you burn during your daily activities. To lose weight, you'll need to create a calorie deficit, in which you take in fewer calories than you expend. In this way, you'll force your body to draw on existing fat stores to meet its energy needs. To do this, you can either eat less food, increase your physical activity, or both. As you'll soon see, a combination of the two is the most effective way to lose weight—and the least painful.

SETTING SENSIBLE GOALS

Before you begin, you'll need to know where you're going and what you hope to accomplish. Start by checking your weight against the Metropolitan Life Insurance Company's height and weight tables. Use the ideal weight in the tables as your ultimate goal. Keep in mind, however, that the tables are less than perfect estimates of the healthiest weights.

Height and weight tables according to frame, ages 25–59: Men.

| Height** | | Weight (lbs)* | | |
Feet	Inches	Small frame	Medium frame	Large frame
5	2	128–134	131–141	138–150
5	3	130–136	133–143	140–153
5	4	132–138	135–145	142–156
5	5	134–140	137–148	144–160
5	6	136–142	139–151	146–164
5	7	138–145	142–154	149–168
5	8	140–148	145–157	152–172
5	9	142–151	148–160	155–176
5	10	144–154	151–163	158–180
5	11	146–157	154–166	161–184
6	0	149–160	157–170	164–188
6	1	152–164	160–174	168–192
6	2	155–168	164–178	172–197
6	3	158–172	167–182	176–202
6	4	162–176	171–187	181–207

*Weight includes indoor clothing weighing 5 pounds for men and 3 pounds for women.
**Height includes shoes with 1-inch heels.
Courtesy Metropolitan Life Insurance Company

Height and weight tables according to frame, ages 25–59: Women.

| Height** | | Weight (lbs)* | | |
Feet Inches	Small frame	Medium frame	Large frame
4 10	102–111	109–121	118–131
4 11	103–113	111–123	120–134
5 0	104–115	113–126	122–137
5 1	106–118	115–129	125–140
5 2	108–121	118–132	128–143
5 3	111–124	121–135	131–147
5 4	114–127	124–138	134–151
5 5	117–130	127–141	137–155
5 6	120–133	130–144	140–159
5 7	123–136	133–147	143–163
5 8	126–139	136–150	146–167
5 9	129–142	139–153	149–170
5 10	132–145	142–156	152–173
5 11	135–148	145–159	155–176
6 0	138–151	148–162	158–179

*Weight includes indoor clothing weighing 5 pounds for men and 3 pounds for women.
**Height includes shoes with 1-inch heels.
Courtesy Metropolitan Life Insurance Company

You may feel fine and look great above the recommended weights. Or you may feel fat at the weight the tables say is ideal for you. Until the medical establishment knows more and can develop individualized goals for each person's ideal weight, the height and weight tables are the best standard we've got.

A weight loss of one to two pounds per week is considered medically safe, and this kind of gradual weight loss is the most successful in the long run. Trying to lose too much weight too quickly can be dangerous to your health. And expecting quick weight loss without being able to achieve it can be discouraging enough to make you go off your diet for good.

To estimate the amount of time it will realistically take to reach your goal, estimate the number of pounds you want to lose and then calculate the number of weeks it will take you to reach the goal if you lose one pound a week. Then do the same calculation using a weight loss of two pounds a week. Mark the dates on a calendar: the time it takes to reach your goal will fall somewhere between these two dates. If you find yourself expecting to reach your goal before that time, you may be setting yourself up for failure.

CUTTING CALORIES

Cutting down on the amount of calories you eat is probably the single most popular way to go about losing weight. Most experts on obesity agree that the most reasonable way to lose weight is a balanced, calorie-restricted diet, one that includes a variety of foods but is limited in calories. Most adults can lose weight on a daily intake of 1,000 to 1,200 calories, although active people or those with a large body frame may need 1,500 to 1,800 calories a day. Anything less than 1,000 calories per day is considered nutritionally inadequate and should only be attempted on your doctor's advice and under his or her supervision.

You'll be pleased to learn that the most effective way to cut back on calories corresponds to the best way to lower your blood cholesterol: by cutting back on the amount of fat you eat. Mounting evidence now suggests that fat is simply more "fattening" than carbohydrates, and that fat calories, more so than total calories, may be the real culprits in contributing to obesity. Remember that fat contains nine calories per gram, compared with four calories per gram of protein or carbohydrate.

But there may be more to dietary fat's role in obesity than just extra calories. Your body converts dietary fat more easily than protein or carbohydrates into body fat. After eating a meal, your body begins the complex chemical process of breaking down the food into a usable form of energy—what's called metabolism. This process itself requires a certain amount of energy. Obesity experts have estimated that your body's energy cost of converting dietary fat to body fat is an extremely efficient 3 percent. The cost of converting carbohydrates to *glycogen,* a type of sugar stored in the muscles, is 7 percent. However, the energy cost of converting carbohydrates to fat is 23 percent. In other words, converting dietary fat to body fat is the easiest thing for your body to do because it requires the least energy; converting carbohydrates to fat is the hardest.

Studies have borne out this biological fact by showing that carbohydrate is only reluctantly turned to fat in the body—and only after study participants eat massive amounts of carbohydrates. (That's not to say you can eat all the carbohydrates you want and not get fat; given enough carbohydrates, your body *will* turn the excess into fat; remember too that you still have to cut calories to lose weight.)

New research on *lipoprotein lipase* (LPL), an enzyme that plays a key role in storing dietary fat in the body's fat tissues, lends more support to the dietary-fat-to-body-fat theory, especially among formerly obese people. In thinner people, levels of LPL drop after a high-fat meal, indicating that the normal body attempts to use fat as energy before storing it as fat. However, when formerly obese women are fed dietary fat, their LPL levels shoot up, suggesting that their bodies are pulling fat calories out for storage.

More evidence that fat calories really are more fattening comes from animal studies. Rats receiving 40 percent of their calories from fat put on twice as much body fat as animals consuming the same calories—or even more—but receiving just 11 percent of those calories from fat. Some studies among men and women showed that the only difference in eating behavior between lean and obese adults was the source of their calories. Surveys and food diaries kept by the study participants showed that lean men and women got about 29 percent of their calories from fat and 53 percent from carbohydrates. Obese volunteers, on the other hand, ate a diet consisting of 35 percent fat and 46 percent carbohydrates.

The complex carbohydrates we recommend that you eat in place of fat, which usually contain a fair amount of dietary fiber, may aid in weight loss by increasing feelings of satiety. High-fiber foods take longer to digest, making you feel full longer, and reducing the temptation to eat foods strictly because you're hungry. (Obviously, high-fiber foods won't change such habits as eating to alleviate stress, which we'll discuss later in this chapter.)

BURNING MORE CALORIES

Some experts say that inactivity, common among overweight people, is a chief cause of obesity. Whether or not that's the case, increased activity factors importantly into the success of any weight-control program.

- Dieting alone can cause you to lose muscle as well as fat. Exercise helps you lose fat while maintaining crucial muscle mass.

- Some studies have shown that dieting alone slows metabolism. Exercise revs up your metabolism, which may stop or reverse this natural response to dieting.

- Contrary to popular belief, exercise doesn't necessarily increase your appetite, which many dieters fear will thwart their weight-loss efforts by causing them to eat more. While marathon runners and other professional athletes consume nearly twice as many calories as sedentary people, they need that many calories just to meet the energy requirements of their training. However, among people who train for relatively short periods of time, exercise doesn't appear to stimulate the appetite or increase food intake.

- If anything, regular exercise may help increase your compliance with your diet. When you exercise while dieting, you won't have to cut calories so severely. This means you won't feel so deprived and will be less likely to go off your diet. In fact, some people may find that if they exercise enough, *they may not have to cut calories from their diet at all.* (You still should cut back on dietary fat, since this raises your blood cholesterol level.) What's more, studies have shown that dieters who exercise are more likely to lose weight and keep it off than those who don't.

- Exercise can help buoy your sense of well-being and increase your confidence.

Many overweight people are discouraged from exercising when they hear they have to expend 3,500 calories to lose just one pound of fat. You can see by checking the calorie expenditure chart in the Appendix that it would take an inordinate amount of exercise to lose one pound: you'd have to play golf for 20 hours, run for 35 miles, or play volleyball for 32 hours. What you may not realize is that unlike exercising for cardiovascular conditioning, which must be performed on a regular basis to do any good, exercising to lose weight is cumulative; that is, you'll lose a pound of fat whether you burn 3,500 calories over the course of a week or over the course of a year—provided your food intake remains fairly constant.

What this means is that for obese people—especially those who lead fairly inactive lives—exercise need not be strenuous to be effective. In fact, even small increases in physical activity help: walking to the store instead of driving your car, for instance.

Of course, by engaging in a regular program of physical activity, you'll be lowering your weight and your risk of heart disease all at once. You'll also lose weight—specifically, body fat—more quickly this way. And, since your body starts drawing on fat reserves after 15 to 30 minutes of strenuous exercise, the longer your exercise session, the

more body fat you'll lose. This is another good reason to
stick with low-impact, low-intensity exercises that can be
sustained for longer periods of time, such as walking.

A NEW WAY OF LIFE

If you've been following the advice in this book to lower
your risk of heart disease, you may have already experienced a drop in your weight—without even trying. If that's
the case, congratulations! Keep up the good work. If you
still don't see a change in your weight, you may have to cut
back on the total amount of food you eat and/or step up your
physical activity a bit more. You may also need to take a
good look at the motivations behind your current eating
and exercise habits. Keep a record for at least two weeks of
what you eat, the time, location, what you are doing and
how you feel when you're eating—without attempting to
change your eating habits just yet. Once you understand
some of your key eating behaviors, you can begin to substitute different ones. For example, instead of eating snacks
in front of the television, try sewing, painting, or writ-
ing letters while watching TV. If you turn to ice cream for
solace after an argument, try doing 10 jumping jacks instead.

You can take the same approach to changing your level
of physical activity. Keep a record of all your daily activities—including such minimal activities as sleeping and eating—for seven days. Then look for ways you can replace
your sedentary ways with physical activity. Get out of your
car, the bus, or train early on your way to work and walk
the remaining distance. Take a walk on your lunch break,
or before work. Or walk up and down several flights of
stairs during your coffee break.

Keeping track of your progress by plotting your weight
changes on a chart helps keep you going, as does giving
yourself encouraging rewards along the way.

MANAGING A CHILD'S WEIGHT

If you're overweight, there's a 40 percent chance that one or more of your children will be overweight. If you and your spouse are both overweight, the likelihood that your progeny will be overweight rises to 80 percent. Without a doubt, obesity is a family affair, due in part to shared genes and in part to a shared life-style.

Keeping your children's weight in check is every bit as important as controlling your own weight. Overweight children as young as five and six have some of the same risk factors for cardiovascular disease as adults, particularly elevated blood pressure and LDL cholesterol. Moreover, overweight children tend to become overweight adults, and these risk factors then become much more dangerous.

But *don't* take your child's weight problems into your own hands. Your pediatrician can judge best whether your child has a weight problem. In children, overweight is determined not so much by the scales as by the fat content of the upper arm, which must be measured with skin fold calipers by a skilled health professional. Your physician can also rule out possible medical causes of obesity, such as the genetic disorder Cushing's syndrome. For this reason, a complete physical examination is recommended before you make any attempts to control a child's weight.

Even if your child is deemed overweight, you should not try to put him or her on a weight-reducing diet without your doctor's advice. Each child's food and energy needs depend on his or her activity level, metabolism, and other factors. And vigorous weight-reducing diets can be dangerous, even causing "stunted" growth.

Your pediatrician may prefer to wait and see if your child will grow out of his or her "baby fat." A balanced, calorie-reduced diet may be recommended for younger children, preteens, or mildly to moderately obese teenagers. This usually involves reducing calories by 25 to 30 percent, mostly by cutting back on fat. Ask your doctor about how many calories your child needs and about safe ways to cut calories in your child's diet—and don't be in a hurry to see results. The rate of weight loss should be even more gradual among children than adults. Most physicians recommend that children lose no more than one to two pounds *every two to four weeks.* Throughout the course of the diet, your child should be carefully monitored by a doctor, who can ensure the child is growing properly.

Watching television appears to be a major contributor to weight problems in children. Among adolescents in one national survey, for each additional hour spent watching TV, the prevalence of obesity increased by 2 percent. Apparently, children are more sedentary when watching TV than when participating in other activities—even such seemingly sedentary activities as reading. They also tend to eat more while watching TV, particularly more of the fat-laden foods advertised on TV.

Substituting almost any other activity for television watching is an improvement. And games and activities that are both fun and require your child to be physically active (such as soccer or bicycling) appear to be best for getting the weight off and keeping it off. Some studies have shown greater and more sustained weight losses among children who participated in a variety of games and other activities as opposed to straight aerobic exercise. Perhaps the most crucial step you can take to help make your child's weight loss effort a success is to get involved yourself. Several studies have shown that parental involvement produces greater and more sustained weight losses than programs aimed only at the child or at parent and child separately.

CHAPTER

6

Managing Stress

YOU have probably heard that the stresses of modern society are a risk factor for heart disease, and that certain personality traits may increase your chances of developing heart disease. You may wonder what to make of all this, and whether your risk is affected by the stresses in your life.

At this point, there seem to be almost as many questions as there are answers about the role of stress in heart disease. Stress is difficult to define, and even more difficult to measure. What stresses some people may exhilarate others. Moreover, we all have our own way of coping with stress, and some coping mechanisms are more constructive than others.

Similar problems exist with research on the coronary-prone *Type A personality*. Experts describe the Type A personality as work-oriented, competitive, aggressive, hostile, easily annoyed when progress is impeded, preoccupied with deadlines, and filled with a chronic sense of time urgency. Of the 31 different characteristics that have been included in descriptions of Type A behavior, only a few key character traits may actually predispose a person to coronary heart disease.

In spite of these problems, there's enough evidence to support the idea of a link between stress and heart disease. The association between the Type A personality and heart disease was so convincing that in 1978, a panel of distinguished biomedical and behavioral scientists convened by the National Heart, Lung, and Blood Institute concluded that "Type A behavior . . . is associated with an increased risk of clinically apparent coronary heart disease in employed, middle-aged U.S. citizens." So it's probably a worthwhile exercise to take stock of the stresses in your life and the way you handle them, as well as certain personality characteristics that may affect your risk of heart disease.

STRESS AND YOUR HEART

Stress is a fact of modern-day life. And it isn't necessarily all bad. Getting married can be just as stressful as getting fired from your job. Dr. Hans Selye, Professor and Director of the Institute of Experimental Medicine and Surgery at the University of Montreal, who has spent nearly 40 years studying the body's physiological response to stress, says everyone needs a little stress to add spice to life.

When scientists talk about stress, they're really referring to *stressors,* events or situations that require you to adapt to your environment in one way or another. A job promotion, for example, demands that you learn and take on new responsibilities. A traffic jam that causes you to miss your plane requires a change in travel plans.

We all respond to feelings of stress in two basic ways: with an *acute reaction,* in which our bodies prepare for quick action against an immediate threat (what's known as the "fight or flight response"), or a *chronic reaction,* which prepares our bodies for long-term endurance. Both stress responses are inborn traits believed to have evolved over millions of years, when early humans had to cope with such physical threats as a saber-toothed tiger in the jungle or a scarcity of food. Both acute and chronic stress responses trigger the release of chemicals from the adrenal glands, located just above the kidneys. These hormones influence the workings of the *sympathetic nervous system,* the part of the central nervous system that governs such involuntary responses as breathing and heart rate.

During acute stress, the adrenal glands churn out *adrenaline (norepinephrine* and *epinephrine).* These two stress hormones accelerate your breathing and heart rate, raise your blood pressure and blood sugar levels, and release high-energy fats into the bloodstream for quick energy. The hormones also increase the "stickiness" of blood platelets, which makes blood clot more easily in case you're wounded.

Chronic stress results in the release of *cortisol,* which causes blood cholesterol levels to rise. Cortisol also causes you to retain sodium, which in turn may increase blood pressure.

These stress responses are well suited for physical threats and a hostile environment: the need to fight off a tiger or run for your life or to go for days or even weeks without food. However, they don't do you much good in dealing with most of today's psychological stressors—traffic jams, long lines, a petulant boss, and such. In fact, the feelings of hopelessness and helplessness that occur when you feel overwhelmed by the stresses in your life may be a real health hazard.

Several studies suggest that the constant firing of the fight or flight response that may result from living in a stressful environment may lead to permanent increases in heart rate and blood pressure. For instance, mice housed in typical laboratory colonies don't develop hypertension. But when they are housed in large groups in a special habitat designed to increase social and territorial confrontations, they develop progressive and eventually irreversible increases in blood pressure.

Studies have also shown increased rates of hypertension among people who have a lot of responsibility but little

control over their environment. Male air traffic controllers
have two to four times the rate of hypertension as men of
similar age in other occupations. Bus drivers also have
higher rates of hypertension, suggesting that high blood
pressure may occur more frequently in jobs that are de-
manding but in which there is little opportunity or flexibility to deal with those demands.

Blood pressure is higher among people of lower socioeconomic status too. Researchers acknowledge that the differences in blood pressure may be related to differences in
diet and exercise habits among people in high and low socioeconomic groups. But they also suggest that the higher
rates of hypertension among these people may be partly
attributed to living in high-crime areas and holding low-
paying (or no) jobs, with little chance of moving up the
socioeconomic ladder.

Cholesterol can also be grossly elevated by stress. In one
study, certified public accountants who were followed from
January 1 to April 15 experienced as much as a 100-mg/dl
rise in cholesterol without a change in their diet. Other
researchers have found that LDL cholesterol is higher and
HDL cholesterol is lower for up to 10 days after an acutely
stressful event. Some animal studies suggest that the chemical changes of the fight or flight response may damage the
lining of the arteries, making it easier for plaques to form
on artery walls. Stress takes its toll in an indirect way as
well. When you become stressed, you may be tempted to
overeat, drink excessive amounts of alcohol, or if you're a
smoker, light up more than usual.

TAKING STOCK OF STRESS

How much stress are you under right now? On a regular
basis? List some of the more stressful situations you now
face—both chronic and acute. Next to each stressful situation, write down ways in which you cope: For instance,
when you're late for an appointment and get stuck in traffic,

do you blow the horn and yell out the window? Reach for a piece of candy to calm your nerves? Light up another cigarette? Turn on the radio and listen to soothing music? Now read the next section to help yourself devise different and perhaps more healthful coping strategies.

ALTERNATIVE WAYS TO MANAGE STRESS

In the last 20 years, much attention has focused on various relaxation techniques—deep breathing, progressive muscular relaxation, several forms of yoga and meditation—and their role in reversing the effects of stress. The techniques help people achieve what Harvard cardiologist Herbert Benson calls the "relaxation response," a state of consciousness marked by decreased oxygen consumption, respiratory rate, heart rate, and blood pressure, and increased activity of slow alpha brain waves. This physiological response is exactly opposite that of the stress-induced fight or flight response.

Relaxation techniques have been found to reduce blood pressure by several points when used in the treatment of hypertension—the higher the blood pressure to begin with, the greater the drop that occurs. Biofeedback, the use of electronic devices to help people influence bodily functions that usually are not under conscious control, has been shown to help keep blood pressure in check for up to six months. Some medicated patients, once trained to lower their blood pressure, can control their blood pressure without medications for up to nine months. Preliminary studies even suggest that long-term use of these procedures may permanently decrease your body's response to the stress hormone norepinephrine.

Volunteers in Dr. Ornish's study actually experienced a reversal of artery narrowing when placed on a strict diet, exercise, and relaxation regimen. While it's not certain just how much of the reversal was due to the stress-reducing techniques, it can't hurt to try.

A PROGRAM TO MANAGE STRESS

A program of stress management doesn't mean you have
to become a Tibetan monk. Practicing relaxation techniques
for just 10 minutes twice a day can make a big difference.
And the only side effects are decreased anxiety and an increased sense of well-being.

There are several relaxation techniques you can use to
manage stress. Dr. Benson's method, described in his book
The Relaxation Response, is among the simplest. To elicit
the relaxation response, follow these steps:

1. Sit quietly in a comfortable position.
2. Close your eyes.
3. Deeply relax all your muscles. (One way to do this is to
   methodically tense and relax each group of muscles in
   your body, beginning with your toes.)
4. Breathe in and out through your nose; repeat the number "one" silently. (This helps clear your mind of extra-
   neous thoughts.)
5. Continue this for 10 to 20 minutes, once or twice daily.
   Maintain a passive attitude during the practice.
6. When finished, sit quietly with your eyes closed for a
   few moments and then gradually open them.

When you find yourself faced with a particularly stressful
situation during the day, such as a nerve-wracking meeting
with your boss, try taking a few deep breaths when you feel
tension mounting. This helps counter the effects of adrenaline. Or try briefly running in place or doing a few jumping
jacks just before or after a stressful event such as a business
meeting or an argument with your spouse. Again, this
helps dissipate the stress hormones by putting them to their
intended use.

Stay away from such stimulants as caffeine and tobacco.
Both intensify the effects of stress on the sympathetic nervous system.

Regular aerobic exercise is another excellent way to relieve stress. If you've begun exercising to keep your heart healthy, you may already feel less stressed and more relaxed.

THE CORONARY-PRONE PERSONALITY

Some people have a characteristic way of responding to environmental stressors, which has become known as Type A behavior or the Type A personality. This cluster of personality traits, including competitiveness, aggression, hostility, impatience, and time urgency, was first described by cardiologists Meyer Friedman and Ray H. Rosenman in the 1974 best-seller *Type A Behavior and Your Heart.* In a study involving some 3,154 men with coronary heart disease, Drs. Friedman and Rosenman reported that Type A men were 2.2 times more likely to develop coronary heart disease than the more relaxed Type Bs.

Over the years, further studies have begun to single out what appears to be one of the most important Type A characteristics associated with an increased heart disease risk: hostility. Several studies have shown that Type A people who become frustrated, irritated, or overreact to trivial events (such as a minor mistake made by a coworker or a long line at the supermarket) are up to five times more likely to develop coronary heart disease than Type A people who don't harbor this kind of free-floating hostility.

ARE YOU A TYPE A PERSONALITY?

Professionals use a rather lengthy questionnaire or interview session to assess Type A behavior. However, there are certain Type A characteristics that you may be able to recognize by yourself. Place a check mark next to the characteristics that best describe you. The more characteristics you mark, the more fully developed is your Type A personality. But checking even one characteristic suggests that you may have some Type A traits.

_____ Do you schedule more activities into your day than you can possibly accomplish?

_____ Do you become easily upset or enraged over minor annoyances, such as waiting in line or driving behind a car you think is moving too slowly?

_____ Do you often find yourself completing the sentences of people you're speaking with?

_____ Are you obsessed with being on time?

_____ Do you become impatient when watching others do things you can do better or faster?

_____ Do you find yourself always competing with or challenging other people, or playing games only to win?

_____ Do you often try to do more than one thing at a time (read a business report while you're eating, or conduct business on your car phone while driving)?

_____ When talking, do you bang your hand on the table or pound one fist into the palm of your hand to make a point?

_____ Do you start feeling guilty when you relax and do nothing for a few days—or even a few hours?

_____ Do you frequently clench your jaw, grit your teeth, tap your fingers, or jiggle your knees?

CHANGING YOUR TYPE A WAYS

In a follow-up study to his research on Type A behavior, Dr. Friedman found that Type A patients could change their coronary-prone behavior. In doing so, they may reduce their risk of a subsequent heart attack. During the five years of the study, those who successfully completed the program of behavior therapy and counseling had fewer recurrences (12.9 percent) than those who received only counseling on diet and exercise (21.2 percent) and those who received no counseling at all (28.2 percent).

Changing your behavior isn't easy. But it may be essential to protect yourself from the ill effects of countless anxiety-producing situations that arise in your life every day. Here are a few suggestions for altering two of the most common traits associated with the Type A personality: hostility and time urgency.

Hostility: Becoming aware of your behavior is the first step toward changing it. Briefly review your list of stressful events and coping mechanisms. If you pound the vending machine when it takes your money or fly off the handle when someone has misplaced the stapler at work, you should rethink the way you deal with these everyday stresses. Keep track of your behavior as you try to make changes for the better. Every day, write down the events that anger or upset you—as soon as you can after the annoying episode. Note how you handled the situation as well. Review your list at the end of each week and ask yourself whether your response was warranted in light of what you now know about free-floating hostility. If you overreacted, write down other, more productive ways in which you could have coped. Doing so will help you get through the next stressful situation.

Time urgency: Many Type As attribute their success in life to getting a lot more done in less time than it takes the average person. However, this scenario can ultimately set you up for failure. Spreading yourself too thin may compromise the quality of your work and can undermine your self-esteem, particularly if you take on too much at one time and can't get it all done. To change your harried ways, start by eliminating some of the activities you can safely do without. Then build in some "idle" time during your day: Make a habit of eating a leisurely breakfast, even if it means getting up a half hour earlier. Take several 10- to 15-minute "do nothing" breaks during the day in which you daydream, meditate, or nap. And make a conscious effort not to do two or more things at the same time.

7

Tobacco, Alcohol, and Your Heart

I F you smoke, the best thing you can do for your heart is to quit. Cigarette smoking is so strongly associated with coronary heart disease that former U.S. Surgeon General C. Everett Koop calls smoking "the most important modifiable risk factor of all." Cigarette smoking is particularly lethal when combined with other risk factors (fig. 5). The good news is that your elevated risk of heart disease begins to decline shortly after you quit smoking.

The role of alcohol in the development of coronary heart disease is much less clear: some studies suggest that a little alcohol may actually protect you. On the other hand, too much alcohol can damage the heart, so prudent use of alcohol is essential.

TOBACCO AND YOUR HEART

Cigarette smoke affects the heart and blood vessels in several ways. When you light up, the nicotine in the smoke increases your blood pressure, heart rate, the amount of blood pumped by your heart, and the blood flow in the coronary arteries. Carbon monoxide in cigarette smoke reduces the amount of oxygen available to your heart and other organs.

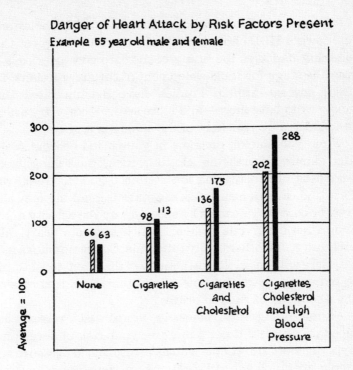

FIGURE 5. Cigarette Smoking and Your Risk of Heart Disease. *This chart shows how cigarette smoking combined with other risk factors (cholesterol levels of 260, systolic blood pressure of 150) affects your risk of suffering a heart attack. For reasons not yet known, the risk of smoking is greater for women than men.* (Reproduced with permission. 1991 Heart and Stroke Facts, 1990. Copyright © American Heart Association.)

Cigarette smoking also raises levels of LDL cholesterol and lowers HDL cholesterol. Animal studies suggest that smoking damages the lining of the coronary arteries, setting the stage for the development of coronary lesions. Indeed, several human studies have demonstrated that smokers do have more—and more severe—coronary artery lesions than nonsmokers of the same sex and age.

When you smoke, platelets in your blood become sticky and cluster, decreasing clotting time, increasing blood thickness, and increasing the likelihood that blood clots will form and cause a heart attack. Cigarette smoking may also trigger coronary spasms by speeding up the activity of the sympathetic nervous system, which controls heart rate, breathing, and other bodily functions. Cigarette smoke may interfere with the electrical activity of the heart, too, leading to irregular heart rhythms (arrhythmias) and increasing the likelihood of sudden death.

Although cigarette smoking *temporarily* raises your blood pressure, it doesn't increase your risk of developing hypertension. But people who have high blood pressure and smoke are much more likely than hypertensive nonsmokers to develop life-threatening *malignant hypertension.*

Women who smoke experience menopause an average of two to three years earlier than nonsmokers. The earlier menopause puts them at increased risk of heart disease because they lose the protective effects of estrogen on the heart (more on that later) much earlier than nonsmokers.

Like many smokers, you may be under the impression that switching to low tar and nicotine cigarettes somehow reduces the smoking-related health risks. However, several studies have shown this just isn't so. In fact, smokers of low tar and nicotine cigarettes often compensate by taking more puffs, taking longer puffs, and inhaling more deeply. Some may even smoke more cigarettes to make up for the lower nicotine content of these brands.

Tobacco's damage to the heart and circulatory system is

not limited to cigarette smoke, either. Even chewing tobacco has been shown to lower HDL cholesterol among teenagers. People who smoke pipes and cigars usually inhale less smoke than cigarette smokers, so their risk of coronary heart disease is lower. However, if you switch from cigarettes to pipes or cigars, you may continue to inhale and your heart disease risk won't be reduced.

Nor do the ill effects of cigarette smoking begin and end with the smoker. When nonsmokers breathe air laced with cigarette smoke even for short periods of time, their blood platelets get sticky, which can help form clots. For nonsmokers with coronary artery disease, this may lead to a heart attack if a clot blocks the heart's blood supply.

Some studies suggest that nonsmoking spouses of cigarette smokers are about 30 percent more likely to suffer from heart disease or to die of a heart attack as a result of exposure to secondhand smoke. Children whose parents smoke have lower HDL cholesterol levels compared with children of the same sex who have nonsmoking parents. When both parents smoke, HDL cholesterol levels are an average 7 percent lower in girls and 4 percent lower in boys.

Calling It Quits

Even if you've smoked virtually all your life, you can substantially reduce your risk of heart disease by quitting now. Within 12 hours after you have your last cigarette, the levels of carbon monoxide and nicotine in your body will be drastically reduced, and your heart and lungs will begin to repair the damage caused by cigarette smoking. Within a few days, your senses of smell and taste will return, and your smoker's hack will disappear. Two years after quitting, your chances of having a heart attack will be cut in half. And ten years after quitting, your risk of dying from heart disease will be almost the same as if you'd never smoked!

You should quit before signs of heart disease appear,

however. Once you develop heart disease, even if you stop smoking, your risk of suffering a heart attack won't return to normal, although it will be lower than if you continue to smoke.

Quitting, of course, may be one of the hardest things you do in your life. Not only do you have to break a physical dependency on nicotine (a drug that may be as addictive as heroin), you also have to change personal habits and rituals. However, withdrawal symptoms—irritability, anxiety, difficulty concentrating, restlessness, headache, drowsiness, and stomach upset—usually subside after a few weeks. And there are several good ways to help you make lasting changes in your personal habits. Remember, too, that as tough as it is to quit now, it's even tougher to deal with the possible health consequences of smoking later on.

Developing a Quit Plan

Some 40 million Americans have already quit smoking. You can too. Here are a few secrets of their success.

Make the decision to quit: Most smokers want to quit. If you're one of them, reinforce your decision by making a list of all the reasons you want to quit. When making your list, don't forget to include your *personal* reasons for wanting to quit, in addition to your health and your obligations to others. Think of all the time and money you use on the habit.

Don't let the fear of gaining weight keep you from quitting. By some estimates, you'd have to put on an additional 75 pounds to offset the health benefits gained by quitting. On average, ex-smokers gain only about five or six pounds. There are several reasons for this. Some studies have found that smoking speeds up your metabolism. When you quit, your metabolism may slow down a little, causing you to gain weight. Still other studies contend that ex-smokers begin to eat more once they quit, which could also explain why they gain weight—but keep in mind that many ex-smokers don't gain any weight at all.

Choose a method: There are several ways to go about quitting. By far the most successful is going it alone. In one of the largest surveys to date on smokers who quit, more than 90 percent did so on their own, without any help from organized smoking cessation programs. And smokers who quit "cold turkey" were more likely to succeed than those who gradually decreased their daily consumption of cigarettes, switched to cigarettes lower in tar or nicotine, or used special filters or holders.

If you decide to go it alone, check out the numerous books, booklets, videotapes, and other materials available to help you. Contact your local chapter of the American Heart Association, American Cancer Society, or American Lung Association for information.

Stop-smoking groups may be helpful for heavier, more addicted smokers who haven't been able to quit on their own. These groups meet at least weekly for about 10 weeks, providing support and helping you find constructive alternatives to smoking. Again, local chapters of the American Heart Association, the American Cancer Society, and the American Lung Association often offer stop-smoking clinics, as do the YMCA, YWCA, and hospitals and health clinics in your area.

Heavy smokers (those who have their first cigarette within 30 minutes after waking up in the morning, or who smoke more than a pack a day) may opt to use nicotine gum or nicotine skin patches. These products help ease physical withdrawal symptoms by keeping some nicotine in the bloodstream. Over the course of the three-month treatment program, you chew fewer and fewer pieces of gum per day, or wear a skin patch containing smaller and smaller doses of nicotine, gradually weaning your body of its addiction to nicotine. At the same time, your physician or a support group helps you overcome your psychological addiction. The gum and skin patches are available by prescription only, and under a doctor's supervision.

Set a date: The most successful ex-smokers set a date for quitting and stop cold turkey on that date. Once you've made the decision to quit, set a quit date about two weeks away and circle the date on your calendar.

Some smokers find it helpful during this time to switch to a brand of cigarettes that's low in tar and nicotine and start to taper down. Others find that switching to a brand of cigarettes they don't like makes it easier to give up smoking.

It's a good idea to start physically conditioning yourself too. Begin a modest exercise regimen, drink more fluids, get plenty of rest, and avoid fatigue. These measures will help you cope with the physical withdrawal symptoms you may experience when you quit.

Know your habit: During the two weeks before you quit, keep a record of when, where, and under what circumstances you light up. This smoker's diary will help familiarize you with your habit and will help you find substitutes for smoking after you quit.

Before your quit date, write down some alternatives to smoking as well. For instance, if you always smoke while driving, plan to take public transportation for a while. Instead of smoking after meals, plan to get up from the table and brush your teeth or go for a walk. This will help you avoid temptation in the days and weeks immediately after quitting.

Call it quits: On the day you quit, throw away all cigarettes and matches. Hide all lighters and ashtrays. You're bound to feel some withdrawal symptoms, such as irritability, anxiety, restlessness, headache, drowsiness, or stomach upset.

To keep your mind occupied and ease some of the withdrawal symptoms, keep very busy. Go to the movies, exercise, take long walks, go bike riding. And buy yourself a treat, or do something special to celebrate. When you get the urge to put something in your mouth, chew gum or munch on crunchy low-fat snacks such as carrot and celery sticks, pickles, or unbuttered popcorn.

Seek out support: Even if you're quitting on your own, you'll need all the support you can get from friends, family, and coworkers. Let them know about your plans to quit and tell them you're counting on them to help reinforce your decision.

Try, try again: Of the 30 percent of smokers who try to quit each year, only about 8 percent are successful. But don't be put off by the high rate of failure. The more times you try, the more likely you will be to succeed. And with every attempt you make, you learn more skills that will eventually get you over the hump. Many ex-smokers try to quit at least two times before they finally stop smoking for good.

ALCOHOL AND YOUR HEART

You may have heard that a drink or two a day keeps heart disease away. Several population studies have suggested that light to moderate drinkers (no more than two drinks per day) have a lower incidence of coronary artery disease than nondrinkers. However, the results of some of these studies have been called into question—most of the studies weren't designed primarily to study the role of alcohol on heart disease, and no one is sure exactly how much alcohol the study participants drank. Most researchers asked participants to tell how much alcohol they consumed without verifying the information with other family members or friends or clinically measuring the amount of alcohol they drank. This method is particularly unreliable among heavy drinkers, which may help explain why there were so few heavy drinkers in the studies.

While the effects of moderate drinking on your risk of heart disease remain uncertain, the effects of heavy drinking are quite clear: high doses of alcohol damage the heart muscle itself, possibly by interfering with protein synthesis essential to keep the muscle tissue healthy. Some alcoholics also suffer a deficiency of the B vitamin thiamine, which damages the heart muscle and eventually leads to heart failure.

Heavy alcohol consumption can also trigger disturbances in heart rhythms. This phenomenon has been dubbed the "holiday heart syndrome" because it occurs more frequently around holidays such as New Year's Eve when alcohol intake is generally highest. Large doses of alcohol dilate the blood vessels in your arms and legs, diminishing the amount of blood returning to the heart and reducing the amount of blood your heart pumps out.

Having even three or four drinks per day increases blood pressure. Some studies suggest that as much as 11 percent of hypertension in men may be attributed to this level of alcohol consumption. Heavy drinking also raises blood triglycerides. In fact, alcohol is second only to diabetes as a cause of high blood lipids among patients who are referred to special lipid clinics. Generally, these people don't respond to dietary or drug treatments unless they limit their alcohol intake.

Until we know more about the possible protective effect of alcohol on heart disease, it's best to limit yourself to no more than two drinks per day. (One drink equals one ounce of hard liquor, four ounces of wine, or 12 ounces of beer.) The benefits of moderate amounts of alcohol—if any—don't increase among people who drink more. In fact, people who have more than three drinks per day are at a sharply increased risk of dying from other diseases.

CHAPTER
8

Other Manageable Risk Factors

Y OUR risk of heart disease can be substantially reduced by controlling two major risk factors: high blood pressure and diabetes mellitus. Women who take estrogens after menopause also appear to prolong their built-in biological protection against coronary heart disease.

HYPERTENSION AND YOUR HEART

As crucial as high blood pressure is in raising your risk of coronary heart disease, we know very little about how hypertension damages the heart and blood vessels. Animal studies have shown that high blood pressure in itself isn't enough to cause narrowing of the coronary arteries. However, when elevated blood pressure is combined with high blood cholesterol levels, hypertension somehow promotes the development of plaques on the arteries. This finding has been borne out by population studies, which show a low incidence of atherosclerosis in hypertensive people with low blood lipid levels. However, the majority of Americans have blood cholesterol levels high enough to set the stage for hypertension to promote atherosclerosis.

Researchers are also finding that many people with

hypertension have elevated levels of a hormone called *atrial natriuretic peptide* (ANP), which plays a role in the excretion of sodium in urine. Preliminary reports suggest that ANP may also help blood platelets aggregate faster, resulting in the formation of blood clots that cause a heart attack or stroke. This finding could help explain why people with high blood pressure are more susceptible to heart attacks and strokes.

Fortunately, hypertension is easily diagnosed and highly treatable. And while doctors have known intuitively that reducing blood pressure reduces the risk of heart disease and stroke, they now have hard evidence. The largest study to date, involving some 37,000 people, shows that for every five to six points that a person's blood pressure is reduced, the risk of heart disease declines by 20 to 25 percent and the risk of stroke by 30 to 40 percent.

Making a Diagnosis

Hypertension is called a "silent killer" because it is virtually symptomless. Many people have high blood pressure for years without knowing it. That's why it's essential to have your blood pressure checked periodically. Most physicians now regularly check your blood pressure every time you visit.

Your doctor takes a blood pressure reading by wrapping an inflatable cuff around your arm, inflating the cuff until blood flow in your arm is temporarily cut off, then gradually loosening the cuff and listening through a stethoscope as blood flow is restored. Blood pressure is measured in *millimeters of mercury,* that is, the amount of pressure needed to raise a column of mercury attached to the cuff. A blood pressure reading consists of two numbers written as a fraction: the top number (also the higher number) represents *systolic,* or contracting, pressure—the force of blood on the arteries as the heart contracts. The bottom number measures *diastolic* pressure, or blood pressure when the heart is at rest. A reading of 120/80 is about normal for most people. And while a rise in either number indicates an increased risk of cardiovascular complications, diastolic pressure is the more sensitive measure of heart disease risk.

If your doctor finds that your blood pressure is elevated during a routine office visit, it doesn't necessarily mean you have high blood pressure. Your blood pressure varies widely over time, depending on many variables, including the activity of your sympathetic nervous system, whether you are sitting or standing, the fluid balance in your body, even your muscle tone. Some 15 percent of people with mildly elevated blood pressure may suffer from "white-coat hypertension," in which their blood pressure is elevated only at the doctor's office. Apparently, the anxiety that often accompanies a visit to the doctor is enough to temporarily raise their blood pressure. If your blood pressure is above 140/90, your doctor will want to measure it again on at least two subsequent visits before making a diagnosis of hypertension.

Most people with elevated blood pressure have what's known as *essential* or *primary hypertension,* which has no known cause. However, about 5 percent of people with high blood pressure have *secondary hypertension*—high blood pressure that is a symptom of an underlying medical problem that, when treated, causes blood pressure to return to normal again. For instance, about 5 percent of women who use oral contraceptives develop high blood pressure, which returns to normal once they stop taking birth control pills. If you are under age 30 and develop high blood pressure, if your blood pressure doesn't fall after drug therapy, or if your blood pressure suddenly worsens, your doctor may look for an underlying cause.

Treating High Blood Pressure

If you have a diastolic blood pressure measurement of 95 or higher, or if your diastolic blood pressure is over 90 and you have other risk factors for cardiovascular disease, including high blood cholesterol, your doctor will recommend antihypertensive treatment. The goal is to get diastolic pressure below 90 with the fewest side effects.

If you have mild hypertension (diastolic blood pressure between 90 and 94) and no other risk factors for cardiovascular disease, your physician will probably recommend that you first try making some changes in your diet and life-style. You may be asked to reduce your sodium intake, lose weight, exercise, control stress, and cut back on alcohol. If you're salt-sensitive, limiting your salt intake to 4 to 6 grams a day (about two teaspoons) may be all you need to do to control your blood pressure.

Common Antihypertensive Medications

If your diastolic blood pressure is higher than 95, or if nondrug therapies fail to lower even mildly elevated blood pressure, your physician may recommend one of several types of antihypertensive drugs to help bring your blood pressure down. Used properly, today's antihypertensive drugs adequately control blood pressure 80 to 90 percent of the time. However, as with any drug therapy, there are side effects. Your physician will try to bring your blood pressure under control with the minimum dose of drugs and the fewest side effects. Remember, though, there is no drug without side effects!

The most commonly prescribed antihypertensive medication, and the one physicians may prescribe first, is a class of drugs called *thiazide diuretics.* These drugs work on the kidneys and rid the body of sodium. Diuretics are cheap, easy to take, and highly effective. However, they may cause an electrolyte imbalance, impotence, and fatigue. More important, diuretics may raise blood sugar and blood cholesterol levels, possibly increasing the risk of coronary heart disease.

Beta blockers, drugs that slow the heart rate and decrease the contracting power of the heart muscle, are commonly prescribed for people with symptoms of coronary heart disease (such as angina pectoris) or people who have had a heart attack. However, these drugs sometimes cause bothersome side effects, including fatigue, impotence, and reductions in HDL cholesterol.

Angiotensin-converting enzyme inhibitors, also known as *ACE inhibitors,* may also be prescribed. These agents are potent dilators of the arteries and veins. In some instances, blood pressure can be markedly lowered with small doses of this class of drugs. ACE inhibitors are also useful for treating heart failure. People who take ACE inhibitors sometimes develop a rash, itching, a cough, or high potassium levels in their blood.

If a single antihypertensive medication fails to lower blood pressure, it may be combined with other drugs.

You may have to visit your doctor as often as once a week when you first start taking your blood pressure medication to ensure that the drug is working properly and that you're not suffering any adverse side effects.

If you have mild hypertension that has been kept in check with drug therapy for at least one year, your physician may gradually reduce the amount of medication you take, particularly if you also have been using nondrug methods (diet, exercise, weight loss) to help control your blood pressure. However, regular medical checkups are a must, since blood pressure can rise again to hypertensive levels even after years without therapy.

DIABETES AND YOUR HEART

Cardiovascular disease is the major cause of death in people who have diabetes, abnormally high blood sugar levels caused by either a lack of insulin or a resistance to insulin. (Insulin is a hormone produced by the pancreas that helps the body's tissues absorb blood sugars and fats.) *Type I (insulin-dependent)* diabetes is the more severe form of the disease. However, people with the milder *Type II (non-insulin-dependent)* diabetes—accounting for 80 to 90 percent of all diabetics—suffer the lion's share of cardiovascular complications.

High blood cholesterol is more common in diabetics, and HDL cholesterol is lower in people with uncontrolled diabetes. High blood sugar levels may also damage the lining of the artery walls, increasing their susceptibility to the formation of plaques. Uncontrolled diabetes may cause blood platelets to stick together more readily, so that blood clots more easily. Diabetes is particularly hard on women, somehow canceling out the protection against heart disease that healthy women enjoy.

Making a Diagnosis

Symptoms of Type I diabetes—excessive hunger and thirst, frequent urination, and weight loss—often appear abruptly and with such severity that a diagnosis is swift and certain. This is not always the case for people with Type II diabetes, however. While some people experience mild symptoms for weeks or months, others may have no symptoms, and the disease can go undetected for years—one reason it is particularly important for people over 40 to have regular medical checkups.

For many people, the first hint that they have Type II diabetes may be increased blood sugar levels in a routine blood or urine test. If you have symptoms (frequent urination, an unquenchable thirst, weight loss, weakness and fatigue, dizziness, headaches, or blurry vision), your physician may recommend that you have a *fasting blood glucose test* or a *glucose tolerance test.* Both tests require that blood be drawn from a vein in your arm after an overnight fast. For the fasting blood glucose test, laboratory technicians will test for high blood sugar levels in a single blood sample. If you take a glucose tolerance test, you'll be given a dose of glucose and you'll have additional blood samples taken at intervals to measure how quickly your body clears the glucose from the bloodstream.

Since the test results can be affected by illness, stress, physical inactivity, weight-loss diets, various drugs, and aging, you may have to take the test more than once before a diagnosis can be made. Fasting blood glucose levels greater than 140 milligrams per deciliter (mg/dl) on at least two separate occasions usually mean that you have diabetes. If you have a glucose tolerance test, you'll be diagnosed as a diabetic if two of the blood samples have glucose levels exceeding 200 mg/dl.

Treating Diabetes

If you're diagnosed with diabetes, you will be working closely with your physician to control it for the rest of your life. Some people have more severe diabetes than others, and only your physician can prescribe a treatment regimen that's right for you.

A cornerstone of therapy for all diabetics is diet. Indeed, many Type II diabetics find that dietary therapy alone can bring the condition under control. However, you should not undertake dietary measures by yourself and should work closely with your doctor and possibly a registered dietitian to develop a diet plan to control your diabetes. Your doctor may recommend that you do the following:

- *Cut back on calories.* If you're overweight (as most Type II diabetics are), you'll be advised to reduce the amount of calories you eat to lose weight. Many Type II diabetics find that simply cutting calories helps lower blood sugar levels, even before they lose weight. Generally, the more recent the onset of Type II diabetes, the more effective weight loss will be.

- *Eat smaller, more frequent meals.* You may be advised to spread out your calories as evenly as possible throughout the day. Eating small meals more frequently during the day keeps you from overwhelming your impaired capacity to metabolize food. (If you're taking insulin, you'll have to plan your meals around your insulin injection.)

- **Eat a balanced, low-fat diet.** Most diabetics are advised to eat a diet that's 50 to 55 percent carbohydrates, 15 percent protein, and 30 to 35 percent fat. Since diabetics are more prone to high cholesterol, saturated fat should constitute just 10 percent of your total daily calories.

Experts once believed that sugar should be avoided altogether because it's rapidly absorbed and sharply raises blood sugar levels. However, when modest amounts of sugar are eaten along with other foods (complex carbohydrates and protein), it doesn't have such a dramatic effect on blood sugar levels. Most physicians now allow up to 5 percent of total carbohydrates as added sugar, provided you eat it with a meal and spread it out throughout the day.

Drugs Used to Treat Diabetes

If you have mild to moderate diabetes and don't respond to dietary therapy, your physician may prescribe oral medications, known as *sulfonylureas,* or *oral hypoglycemic agents,* to help lower your blood sugar levels. There are several different kinds of sulfonylureas, but most differ only in their potency and in how often you must take them each day. The major drawback to these drugs is that they sometimes cause *hypoglycemia,* low blood sugar levels that trigger such symptoms as sweating, shakiness, anxiety, heart palpitations, and weakness. Serious episodes of hypoglycemia may result in confusion, irritability, abnormal behavior, convulsions, coma, and in rare instances, death. Most cases of hypoglycemia can be quickly brought under control. Your doctor will tell you how.

Your physician will start you on a low dose of sulfonylureas and gradually increase the dosage until your blood glucose levels return to normal or until the maximum dosage is given. Often, if one drug doesn't work, another will.

About 10 to 20 percent of Type II diabetics don't respond to oral medications. Others may find that these drugs work well for a year or two, then stop working. For these people, as well as Type I and Type II diabetics who have high blood sugar levels (more than 230 mg/dl), insulin injections are necessary.

How much insulin you take and how often depends on the type of insulin you take: the various insulin preparations differ in the amount of time it takes them to start working, the degree of purity, and the source (beef, pork, beef-pork, or human synthetic insulin). Your insulin needs will also depend on your individual reaction to the drug. Some people have higher levels of circulating anti-insulin antibodies, others may not readily absorb the drug. Even your level of physical activity affects your insulin requirement. Many Type II diabetics can control their blood sugar levels with a single daily injection. As with oral medications, the biggest problem with insulin therapy is that it sometimes triggers episodes of hypoglycemia. Even the most rigorous insulin therapy can't match the body's fine-tuned system of keeping blood sugar within its narrowly defined limits.

HORMONES AND YOUR HEART

Experts have long suspected that the reproductive hormones *estrogen* and *progesterone* influence a woman's risk of heart disease. Estrogen, in particular, is believed to somehow protect against heart disease. Postmenopausal women, whose estrogen levels are low, are more than twice as likely to develop heart disease as premenopausal women. But studies now show that postmenopausal women who take estrogens to help control hot flashes and protect against the bone-thinning disorder osteoporosis *have about half the number of heart attacks as women not using hormones.* In one of the best-designed studies to date, the Nurses' Health Study, involving some 48,000 women, Dr. Meir J. Stampfer and colleagues at the Harvard School of Medicine found that those who took postmenopausal estrogens were 50 percent less likely to suffer a heart attack than nonusers. Estrogen users had no greater risk of stroke than nonusers, either. No one is sure yet just how estrogen protects. We do know, however, that natural estrogens given to postmenopausal women lower LDL cholesterol from 5 to 10 percent and raise protective HDL cholesterol from 10 to 15 percent. Estrogen may guard against coronary heart disease in another way, as well. Animal studies and research on women who have had heart surgery suggest that estrogens somehow prevent the formation of fatty deposits on the artery walls.

Progesterone is a different story. Synthetic progestins are typically given along with postmenopausal estrogens to reduce the risk of endometrial cancer. But progestins blunt estrogen's effects on HDL cholesterol. The hormones also increase blood sugar levels. Whether these changes are enough to cancel out estrogen's protective effect is still not known. (A major multicenter study—the Postmenopausal Estrogen/Progestin Interventions Trial, or PEPI—is under way to determine the effects of various combinations of these hormones on a woman's risk of coronary heart disease.)

Should postmenopausal women take hormone replacement therapy (HRT) to protect themselves against heart disease? If you are at high risk for heart disease, you may want to consider taking HRT. A growing number of experts now feel that the benefits of taking estrogens to protect against heart disease far outweigh the only slightly increased risk of breast cancer associated with postmenopausal estrogens. (If you have a high risk for breast cancer, it's probably better not to take HRT.) Discuss the benefits and risks of postmenopausal estrogens with your doctor. Then decide.

On the other hand, women of childbearing age who take

oral contraceptives have two times the heart attack risk of women who don't. For healthy women, this increased risk doesn't pose a problem, because a woman's risk is so low to begin with. But when combined with other risk factors, such as cigarette smoking, the risk rises dramatically. If you have high blood cholesterol, high blood pressure, or other risk factors for heart disease, you should consider using another form of contraception.

It may seem contradictory that menopausal estrogen therapy can protect women against heart disease while the estrogen in oral contraceptives increases the risk of heart disease and stroke. We're still not sure why this is so. One reason may be that the estrogen used after menopause is given in much lower doses than the estrogen in oral contraceptives. High doses of estrogen may cause the blood to clot more easily in susceptible women, and thus increase the risk of heart disease.

Oral contraceptives also contain high doses of synthetic progestins, hormones that increase LDL cholesterol, decrease HDL cholesterol, and increase blood sugar levels, all of which raise your risk of heart disease.

Some women also develop hypertension as a result of taking birth control pills. Blood pressure returns to normal after pill use is discontinued, however.

Most of the information we have about the Pill was obtained years ago when high doses of estrogen were used. The newer, low-dose oral contraceptives are believed to be much safer. Some preliminary evidence even suggests that the risk of heart attack is not increased unless a woman smokes or has other coronary risk factors.

We do know, however, that once you stop taking birth control pills, you aren't at any additional risk of developing heart disease. Recent studies have shown that even women who took oral contraceptives for up to 10 years are at no greater risk of heart disease after they stop taking the Pill than women who never took oral contraceptives.

CHAPTER

9

How Your Doctor Can Help

WHEN life-style measures fail to reduce your cholesterol to safer levels, your physician has an arsenal of highly effective medications to do the job. The most widely prescribed drugs lower LDL cholesterol by an average of 25 to 30 percent. Some of the newer medications are easier to take and have fewer side effects than the standard remedies. More good news: several studies now show that drug therapy combined with a low-fat diet can actually reverse the accumulation of artery-clogging plaques.

WHEN DRUG THERAPY IS RECOMMENDED

If changes in your diet and life-style fail to significantly reduce your cholesterol after six months, your doctor may recommend drug therapy. Generally speaking, men whose LDL cholesterol levels are between 160 and 190 mg/dl after six months of dietary therapy should begin drug therapy if they have at least one other risk factor for heart disease. Women may receive cholesterol-lowering medication if their LDL cholesterol levels remain between 160 and 190 mg/dl after six months on a low-fat diet and they have at least two other risk factors for heart disease.

There are several types of cholesterol-lowering drugs;

each works in a different way. All medications must be used in conjunction with a low-fat diet, and all have side effects.

Bile Acid Sequestrants

These drugs (also known as *resins*) have one of the best track records for reducing the risk of coronary heart disease and are safe enough even for children and for women considering pregnancy. The two sequestrants available today, *cholestyramine* and *colestipol,* are powders that must be mixed with water or fruit juice and taken with meals. Both drugs work by preventing bile acids in the intestine from circulating in the bloodstream. This causes the liver to dip into its cholesterol stores and produce more bile acids, which the body needs to help break down fats. As the liver's cholesterol reserves are depleted, the LDL receptors in the liver step up their activity, taking LDL cholesterol from the bloodstream and thus reducing blood cholesterol levels. When used regularly, bile acid sequestrants lower LDL cholesterol from 15 to 30 percent.

Since bile acid sequestrants aren't absorbed by the gastrointestinal tract, they're extremely safe. However, the drugs commonly cause bothersome side effects, including constipation, bloating, nausea, and gas. Many people find the resins messy and inconvenient to take. Another problem with bile acid sequestrants is that they often raise blood triglyceride levels. For this reason, people with high blood cholesterol *and* high triglycerides are usually given a different medication.

Nicotinic Acid

A prescription form of the water-soluble B vitamin niacin (also known as *nicotinic acid*) has been used to safely lower blood lipid levels for many years. Niacin decreases the liver's production of VLDL cholesterol, which in turn lowers LDL cholesterol in the bloodstream. Some studies have shown that nicotinic acid lowers total cholesterol by up to

25 percent. Nicotinic acid also raises levels of protective HDL cholesterol.

Nicotinic acid is inexpensive and highly effective in reducing cholesterol levels. It's convenient as well: many patients can take a single daily dose of 1.5 to 2 grams of niacin after dinner. However, niacin causes a number of bothersome side effects that make it unacceptable for some people. The most common side effect is *flushing* (reddening of the skin and heat sensations). Most people build up a tolerance to flushing after taking the drug for several weeks. Flushing is less bothersome if you take smaller doses (100 to 250 milligrams) when you first start therapy and gradually increase the dosage over the course of a week or two. Taking your medication on a full stomach reduces flushing as well. Some people find that taking aspirin or nonsteroidal anti-inflammatory drugs (such as ibuprofen) an hour or so before taking niacin also helps control flushing.

Nicotinic acid may occasionally raise levels of blood sugar and uric acid (a by-product of protein metabolism). Niacin sometimes causes nausea, diarrhea, and heart palpitations. Liver toxicity may be a problem when niacin is taken in large doses or in a time-released form. For these reasons, your physician may perform tests of liver function, blood glucose and uric acid levels before beginning a regimen of nicotinic acid and again after you've started therapy. This is also why *you should not attempt to treat yourself with over-the-counter niacin.* Your doctor will recommend another type of medication if you have a peptic ulcer, liver disease, or gout (a condition caused by high levels of uric acid), all of which nicotinic acid can aggravate.

HMG CoA Reductase Inhibitors

One of the most exciting recent advances in the treatment of elevated LDL cholesterol has been the discovery of drugs that inhibit the enzyme *HMG CoA reductase,* a key enzyme in the liver's production of cholesterol. Several of these drugs, called HMG CoA reductase inhibitors, are now being evaluated, including *lovastatin, simvastatin,* and *pravastatin.* So far, only lovastatin has been tested extensively in humans and has been approved by the U.S. Food and Drug Administration for the treatment of elevated cholesterol.

There's plenty of reason for excitement: Lovastatin comes in the form of a pill that can be conveniently taken once daily with dinner. And side effects (including constipation, diarrhea, upset stomach, gas, headaches, fatigue, skin rashes, and muscle weakness) are uncommon, occurring in only about 5 percent of patients who take the drug. Lovastatin is highly effective as well; short-term studies have shown that the drug reduces LDL cholesterol from 25 to 45 percent.

Studies are now under way to determine whether there are any long-term side effects associated with the drug. For now, however, lovastatin is generally prescribed for people at greatest risk of developing coronary heart disease and for patients with known coronary artery disease and elevated cholesterol.

Other Drugs

Several additional drugs may also be prescribed to help keep cholesterol in check, either by themselves or in combination with other cholesterol-lowering drugs.

Fibric acids: These drugs have been used to lower blood triglyceride levels for the past 30 years. The two FDA-approved drugs, *gemfibrozil* and *clofibrate,* are primarily used to reduce the risk of *pancreatitis* (inflammation of the pancreas) among people with high blood triglycerides. Nevertheless, studies have shown that gemfibrozil is safe and effective for reducing the risk of coronary heart disease as well.

Fibric acids appear to enhance the activity of *lipoprotein lipase,* an enzyme that helps break down fats in the bloodstream. Gemfibrozil, the more widely used of the two approved fibric acids, lowers triglycerides and raises HDL cholesterol. It is sometimes prescribed for patients who don't tolerate the resins or nicotinic acid, or in combination with other cholesterol-lowering drugs. Common side effects include a variety of gastrointestinal symptoms, including upset stomach and abdominal pain, and abnormalities in liver function tests.

Clofibrate, which has about the same effect on blood lipids as gemfibrozil and similar side effects, is prescribed less often because long-term use of the drug has been associated with the formation of gallstones and inflammation of the gallbladder.

Probucol: This drug, which increases the rate at which the liver breaks down LDL cholesterol, reduces LDL cholesterol by 8 to 15 percent. Probucol also helps reduce the size of *xanthomas,* cholesterol-filled plaques that sometimes build up on the tendons of people with FH. However, probucol also reduces HDL cholesterol by up to 25 percent, making its role in the treatment of high LDL cholesterol uncertain.

On the other hand, probucol may protect against heart disease in another way. This drug is a powerful *antioxidant* that apparently prevents LDL cholesterol from becoming oxidized, a chemical process in which an oxygen molecule combines with (and damages) the lipoprotein. Some studies now suggest that oxidation of LDL cholesterol within the artery wall may be a critical step in the development of artery-narrowing plaques.

Combined Drug Treatment

If your condition does not substantially improve with single-drug therapy, your physician may combine your medication with another cholesterol-lowering drug to increase its effectiveness. When bile acid sequestrants are combined with either nicotinic acid or lovastatin, the combination appears to reduce blood cholesterol levels much more than either drug taken alone. For instance, in one study when lovastatin was combined with colestipol, the two drugs reduced LDL cholesterol by about 53 percent. Lovastatin alone decreased the level of LDL cholesterol by only 34 percent. A few studies now show that combined drug therapy also can reverse the progression of plaque buildup in the coronary arteries.

People who took a combination of medications didn't suffer any serious side effects either. The most bothersome side effects in these studies were usually related to niacin. Scientists are still investigating the safety and effectiveness of other drug combinations, such as lovastatin and niacin.

OTHER APPROACHES

The majority of people with high blood cholesterol usually see a significant reduction in their cholesterol levels after taking one or more of the medications now available. Sometimes, however, more drastic measures may be needed. For instance, some people with familial hypercholesterolemia may undergo *plasmapheresis,* in which a portion of blood plasma is withdrawn from the body, some of the LDL cholesterol is removed, and the treated blood plasma is then reinjected into the patient's bloodstream. A surgical procedure, *partial ileal bypass,* in which part of the intestine responsible for the absorption of cholesterol is bypassed, occasionally has been used to lower LDL cholesterol in people with heterozygous FH. However, diet and drugs usually reduce cholesterol better than surgery, and with fewer complications.

Liver transplants have been used to treat people with homozygous FH and are highly effective. However, the procedure is rather drastic, requiring patients to take antirejection drugs for the rest of their lives. At this point, no one knows how effective liver transplants will be over long periods of time.

TREATING CHILDREN WITH DRUGS

As you have already seen, there are still many more questions than answers about how best to treat high blood cholesterol in children. While studies have found evidence of fatty streaks in the arteries of children as young as age 10, no one is sure yet how old a child should be before beginning drug therapy. Few studies have been conducted to show which drugs or drug combinations are most effective or how safe these medications are when taken for long periods of time. There's doubt, too, about how much to reduce a child's blood cholesterol levels and whether treating high cholesterol in children will lower the risk of coronary heart disease later in life.

Right now, *no* cholesterol-lowering medications have been approved by the U.S. Food and Drug Administration for use in children. Nevertheless, drug therapy may be prescribed for some children with familial hypercholesterolemia. Typically, these children are given bile acid sequestrants to help lower their blood cholesterol levels. As you may recall, these drugs are not absorbed by the gastrointestinal tract, so the risk of toxicity is very low. But the drugs' side effects, particularly gastrointestinal upsets, are not always easy for children to handle. Ongoing studies are investigating the safety and effectiveness of combinations of drugs, including bile acid sequestrants teamed up with either lovastatin or niacin.

WHAT ABOUT ASPIRIN?

Aspirin doesn't lower blood cholesterol, but it does keep clot-forming blood platelets from building up, thereby helping to prevent blood clots that often cause heart attacks. One major study, the Physician's Health Study, conducted at Harvard Medical School and Brigham and Women's Hospital in Boston, found that the risk of a first heart attack was reduced by 14 percent among men who took an aspirin every other day during the four-year study. A British study, however, found no evidence that aspirin protects against the risk of heart attack. And in both studies, aspirin-takers suffered more strokes from *cerebral hemorrhage* (bleeding from a ruptured blood vessel in the brain) than men who took a placebo.

Should you regularly take aspirin to prevent a heart attack? Not without first discussing it with your doctor. Aspirin, readily available over the counter, is not safe for everybody. If you have liver or kidney disease, a peptic ulcer, gastrointestinal bleeding, or other bleeding problems, you may not be able to take aspirin at all, or you may need to adjust the amount you take. The drug prolongs bleeding, so your doctor should be notified that you're taking aspirin if you're going to have surgery. Also, if you have uncontrolled hypertension or any condition that might increase the risk of a stroke, you should not take aspirin routinely without first checking with your physician. Remember, too, that taking aspirin is just one of several tools you have to reduce your risk of a heart attack. It should be used *in addition to* other preventive measures, such as a low-fat diet and exercise, not as a substitute for these heart-healthy habits.

WHEN HEART TROUBLE HITS

Prevention is the best medicine, and making life-style changes now can significantly reduce your odds of having a heart attack later on. However, preventive measures can't guarantee that you won't develop heart problems.

Fortunately, life-style changes and treatment advances in the last 10 to 15 years have vastly improved the outlook for people who suffer a heart attack: of the estimate 1.5 million Americans who have a heart attack today, *roughly two-thirds will survive.*

One key to survival is to *seek medical help at the first signs of heart trouble*. Here are a few symptoms to watch out for:

Angina pectoris: Discomfort in the chest, often described as a feeling of pressure or tightness lasting several minutes and often triggered by physical exertion, exposure to cold, or stress. If you have an angina attack, you should notify your physician as soon as possible. Your physician may want to perform a few diagnostic tests, such as an electrocardiogram, an exercise stress test, or a coronary angiogram, and may also prescribe drugs to see if the angina can be controlled. Commonly used drugs are *nitrates* (nitroglycerin) and *calcium antagonists* (also known as calcium channel blockers), which help dilate the coronary arteries, and beta blockers, which slow the heart rate and decrease the contracting power of the heart muscle.

Heart attack: If you're at increased risk of developing coronary heart disease, it's imperative that you know the warning signs of a heart attack. *You should immediately call for emergency help if you experience*

- an uncomfortable pressure, fullness, squeezing, or pain in the center of the chest that does not go away in a few minutes
- severe chest pain
- pain spreading to the shoulders, neck, or arms
- lightheadedness and palpitations
- fainting
- sweating associated with chest discomfort
- nausea associated with chest discomfort
- difficulty breathing

Prompt medical attention may reduce the damage to your heart, and the more quickly you receive medical care, the greater are your chances of surviving the heart attack.

CHAPTER

10

A Glimpse into the Future

THE day may come when gene therapy can permanently cure people with inherited illnesses.

That day may be closer than you think. Already, researchers at the University of Michigan in Ann Arbor plan to test a new type of gene therapy in people afflicted with the most severe form of familial hypercholesterolemia, homozygous FH. The treatment involves surgically removing about 15 percent of the patient's liver, isolating certain cells from the tissue, and inserting into the cells a copy of the gene that produces LDL receptors. The treated liver cells are then reintroduced into the patient's body through a small vein that feeds into the liver. If all goes as expected, the treated cells will take up residence in the liver and begin producing LDL receptors to clear excess LDL cholesterol from the bloodstream. The researchers don't know yet how long the therapeutic effects will last, however.

This and other experiments now under way mark the start of a new era in medicine. Already, children afflicted with a rare and devastating immune disorder called *severe combined immunodeficiency* (SCID) are receiving gene therapy to correct a deficiency in an enzyme called *adenosine deaminase* (ADA), which breaks down damaging

by-products of the body that can destroy immune cells. By
the turn of the century, geneticists will have mapped nearly
the entire sequence of 50,000 to 100,000 genes that make
up the human genome. The knowledge gleaned from this
project holds the hope of a cure for any number of illnesses,
including familial hypercholesterolemia and other inherited forms of high blood cholesterol.

The concept behind gene therapy is simple enough: insert
a healthy gene into a patient to take the place of a defective
gene that's causing an inherited illness. But the genetic
code that makes us human is extremely complex. Up to
100,000 genes, tucked away in the nucleus of every cell in
your body, contain the complete chemical instructions for
making a human being. These genes are situated on 23
pairs of chromosomes (one set of 23 chromosomes inherited
from your mother, the other from your father), consisting
of a long, double strand of DNA that twists around like a
spiral staircase. Each gene contains the code for producing
a single *polypeptide,* the building blocks for the proteins
that make up the human body.

Even a minor defect in a gene can throw off protein production and result in illness. So far, nearly 5,000 inherited
conditions caused by single-gene defects have been cataloged. And new ones are being added every week, thanks
to new technology that now is helping to map the entire
human genome at breakneck speed. Countless more inherited conditions involve more than one gene or a combination
of genes and environment.

Once a gene has been found, scientists can more easily
track down the protein for which it codes. The hope is that
by replacing the defective gene with a gene containing the
correct protein code, certain inherited disorders can be
cured. Single-gene disorders hold the most promise for
gene therapy, since they require manipulation of only one
gene. And autosomal conditions resulting in a deficiency
of a certain protein (such as SCID and the LDL receptor

deficiency of heterozygous FH) will be easier to treat than those in which the body produces an excess amount of a protein. Still, many obstacles must be overcome before gene therapy becomes a standard treatment—and even more roadblocks stand in the way before gene therapy can offer a permanent cure.

Essentially, geneticists can treat either *germ cells* (sperm, eggs, or early embryos) or *somatic cells* (any of the rest of the cells in your body). Both types of cells contain a complete set of genes. However, unlike somatic cells, germ cells have the unique ability to pass on the genetic code to all the other cells in your body. Germ cells can also pass on one copy of genetic instructions to another germ cell—which is what happens when a sperm cell and egg cell join.

Successfully treating germ cells in the early stages of life could conceivably cure an affected person and all of his or her offspring. But the practice raises profound ethical questions: within a generation or two, we could permanently alter the gene pool of the human race—possibly in ways that would be detrimental to our survival as a species. We'd also be tampering with millions of years of evolution. And there's always the possibility of abuse: Would gene therapy be used simply to correct an inherited illness, or would it also be used to improve our offspring by engineering "super genes" for a "master race"?

Fortunately, many inherited illnesses are caused by a flaw in specialized cells or parts of cells—such as defective LDL receptors in people with familial hypercholesterolemia—so it's not necessary for *all* of the body's 75 trillion cells to contain the correct copy of a gene. This makes it possible to treat many inherited illnesses by manipulating somatic cells. And since this type of gene therapy affects only the treated individual, the ethical issues are much less controversial.

Treating somatic cells has its own unique set of problems, however. For instance, specialists have been grappling with the question of how to get a copy of the new gene into *only* those cells affected by the genetic flaw. It's not possible simply to inject foreign genes into the bloodstream and expect them to home in on target cells and take over. To begin with, your immune system would quickly recognize the new DNA as a foreign invader and attack and destroy it. Even if the foreign DNA wasn't destroyed by your immune cells, there's no guarantee that it would reach the cells it was intended to treat.

Geneticists have tried splicing the new gene directly into a cell's nucleus, but this process is extremely inefficient. For every gene spliced in the correct place, more than 1,000 slip into other parts of the DNA.

Now, however, researchers have found an ingenious and highly effective way to replace defective genes with new ones through the use of *retroviruses.* Normally, these virus cells sneak into your own cells undetected by your immune defense system. Once inside, the virus replaces the cell's healthy DNA with its own viral DNA, which can result in a variety of illnesses. Acquired immune deficiency syndrome (AIDS), for instance, is believed to be caused by a retrovirus.

However, in gene therapy, the disease-causing viral DNA is crippled so that it is incapable of reproducing. Then the cell's nucleus is injected with DNA containing a correct version of the gene being targeted for treatment. The re-engineered viruses are placed in a culture dish along with cells containing the defective gene. The viral cells quickly infiltrate the target cells, replacing the flawed gene with a healthy one.

Obviously this technique works best with cells that can be easily removed from the body, grown in a culture dish, and reintroduced back into the body without being damaged. The treated cells must also have the capacity to reproduce fairly rapidly, so a large colony of new cells containing the healthy gene can be established. Some of the body's cells—neurons in the brain, for instance—reproduce very slowly, if at all, in a person's lifetime and are not good candidates for this type of gene therapy. On the other hand, skin, blood, and liver cells are some of the fastest dividing cells, producing a fresh batch within a few weeks or months. And these cells are fairly accessible, making them prime candidates for gene therapy. This is good news for people with genetically linked lipid disorders, since the liver plays a crucial role in the processing and disposal of cholesterol and other blood fats.

The University of Michigan researchers are particularly hopeful that gene therapy for people with familial hypercholesterolemia will work because animal studies have already shown that liver cells can be genetically retooled to produce more LDL receptors. One experimental procedure involved a strain of rabbits that, like humans afflicted with FH, have a genetic deficiency of LDL receptors. Liver cells were surgically removed from the rabbits, and the gene for LDL receptors was inserted into the cells in a culture dish. As expected, the cells began producing more active receptors—for a while.

Researchers are now experimenting with an LDL receptor gene packaged within a protein carrier that homes to the liver. The encoded gene is injected into the animals' bloodstreams, where the protein makes a beeline for the liver, depositing the new gene inside the liver cells. The hope is that the treated cells will start producing active LDL receptors. In humans, this kind of procedure would eliminate the need for surgery to remove liver cells. The procedure has met with some measure of success: the encoded protein was detected in the treated rabbits—but only for a short time.

And herein lies the other major obstacle in treating somatic cells: the types of cells that are most easily treated with today's technology often aren't terribly long-lived in the body. After the genetically engineered cells die, the inherited condition begins to express itself again—unless the patient continues to receive treatment.

There's hope that in the years ahead work on the Human Genome Project will help overcome some of these problems. Essentially, researchers are trying to decipher the genetic code in an estimated 3 billion DNA fragments within each of our cells.

Once the human genome has been entirely mapped out, we'll have the information at hand to break the genetic code for any number of inherited conditions, including hypertension, diabetes, obesity, and the numerous genetic causes of high blood cholesterol and atherosclerosis.

It may be years before gene therapy offers up a permanent, onetime cure for inherited illnesses. However, our new knowledge will give us a much better understanding of the way many of these conditions develop. This, in turn, should lead to more effective treatments and better means of prevention for people at risk of developing heart disease. In effect, the chances of beating the odds against heart disease are improving every day.

Glossary

Angina pectoris: A discomfort in the chest caused by reduced blood flow to the heart muscle. Angina is usually triggered by exercise, exposure to cold, or stress, and is often relieved by rest and relaxation.

Angiography: An X-ray examination of the coronary blood vessels in which a fluid is injected into the bloodstream and X rays are taken as the fluid passes through the coronary arteries.

Angiotensin-converting enzyme (ACE) inhibitors: These drugs are potent dilators of the arteries and veins, and are generally prescribed to lower blood pressure and increase the output of blood flowing from the heart.

Apolipoprotein: The protein part of lipoproteins that is responsible for transporting fat and cholesterol through the body. *See also* Lipoproteins.

Arrhythmias: Irregular heart rhythms.

Arteriosclerosis: A disorder of the arteries associated with advancing age and certain diseases (notably hypertension) in which the connective tissues in the artery walls become stiffer and less elastic. This results in decreased blood flow, especially to the brain and extremities.

Atherosclerosis: Progressive narrowing of the coronary arteries due to the buildup of *plaques* (consisting of cholesterol, fat, and other substances) along the inner walls of the arteries.

Atrial natriuretic peptide (ANP): A hormone that plays a role in the excretion of sodium in the urine. Preliminary reports suggest the hormone may also affect blood-clotting substances (platelets), making them aggregate faster and promoting the development of blood clots. Many people with high blood pressure have elevated levels of ANP.

Autosomal dominant trait: An inherited characteristic, such as brown hair, in which only one gene is needed for the trait to be expressed.

Autosomal recessive trait: An inherited characteristic in which two copies of a gene—one from each parent—are required for the trait to be expressed. People with blue eyes inherit a gene coding for blue eyes from each parent.

Balloon angioplasty: A procedure in which a small balloon is inserted through a catheter into a coronary artery and inflated to unblock the artery.

Beta blockers: Drugs that slow the heart rate and decrease the contracting power of the heart muscle. Beta blockers are typically prescribed for the treatment of hypertension and angina.

Bile acids: These acids are made by the liver and take up residence in the small intestine, where their job is to help in the digestion and absorption of dietary fat and cholesterol.

Bile acid sequestrants: A class of drugs (also known as *resins*) used to lower blood cholesterol levels. The drugs prevent bile acids in the intestines from circulating in the bloodstream. As a result, the liver makes more bile acids from cholesterol stores in the liver. As the liver's cholesterol reserves are reduced, LDL receptors in the liver become more active, taking LDL cholesterol from the bloodstream and thus reducing LDL cholesterol levels in the blood.

Blood pressure: The force exerted by blood on the artery walls as the heart beats. A blood pressure measurement consists of two numbers written as a fraction: the top number, or *systolic pressure,* is the force of blood against the artery walls as the heart contracts; the bottom number, or *diastolic pressure,* reflects blood pressure on the artery walls between heartbeats as the heart relaxes.

Calcium antagonists: These drugs, also known as *calcium channel blockers,* dilate the coronary arteries by blocking the entry of calcium into the smooth muscle tissues of the heart and arteries. Calcium antagonists are prescribed to help control angina and to treat other heart conditions such as arrhythmias and hypertension.

Cardiovascular disease: Any of a number of illnesses affecting the heart and blood vessels, including coronary heart disease, high blood pressure, and stroke.

Cerebral hemorrhage: A type of stroke that occurs when a blood vessel in the brain breaks and results in excessive bleeding.

Cholesterol: A complex chemical found in all animal fats and in every cell in your body. Cholesterol plays a key role in the formation of cell membranes and also helps in the manufacture of certain hormones.

Cholestyramine: One of two types of *bile acid sequestrants,* a class of drugs used to lower blood cholesterol levels. Colestipol is the other type of bile acid sequestrant commonly prescribed. *See also* Bile acid sequestrants.

Chromosomes: Threadlike structures in the nucleus of every cell that carry genes. Chromosomes are composed of a twisting strand of DNA (*deoxyribonucleic acid*) containing the genes, and protein. Most human cells contain 46 chromosomes: 22 pairs of homologous chromosomes and one pair of sex chromosomes. One set of 23 chromosomes is inherited from each parent.

Colestipol: One of two types of *bile acid sequestrants,* a class of drugs used to lower blood cholesterol levels. Cholestyramine is the other type of bile acid sequestrant commonly prescribed. *See also* Bile acid sequestrants.

Coronary heart disease: A form of cardiovascular disease that occurs when deposits of fat and scar tissue (plaques) gradually build up on the inner walls of the coronary arteries, the blood vessels that supply nutrients and oxygen to the heart muscle. This may result in reduced or even blocked blood flow to the heart.

Coronary thrombosis: A blood clot that forms in the coronary arteries, which usually results in a heart attack.

Cystic fibrosis: An inherited disorder in which the body's glands—particularly those of the pancreas, lungs, and intestines—become clogged with thick mucus. Cystic fibrosis is the most common fatal genetic disease among young Americans.

Diabetes mellitus: Abnormally high blood sugar levels caused when the body either doesn't produce enough of the pancreatic hormone *insulin* or is unable to use insulin efficiently. There are two forms: Type I (insulin-dependent) diabetes usually develops before age 25. People with this disorder produce very little insulin and must take insulin injections to control blood sugar levels. Type II, or non-insulin-dependent diabetes, typically develops in adulthood (after age 40). In many Type II diabetics, the pancreas produces insulin, but the body somehow becomes resistant to insulin's effects on blood sugar. Type II diabetes can often be controlled through dietary and weight-loss measures.

Diastolic blood pressure: *See* Blood pressure.

Dietary fiber: The indigestible part of plant foods. There are two types: (1) *water-insoluble fiber,* which doesn't dissolve in water and is found mostly in wheat bran and whole-wheat products, and (2), *water-soluble fiber,* which dissolves in water and forms a gummy gel. Foods

high in soluble fiber include oat bran, fruits and vegetables, and dried peas and beans.

DNA (deoxyribonucleic acid): The genetic material within
the nucleus of every cell containing 23 pairs of chromosomes and some 50,000 to 100,000 genes.

Echocardiography: A diagnostic test in which high-
frequency sound waves (ultrasound) are used to see the
structure of the heart.

Electrocardiogram (ECG): A diagnostic test that measures
the heart's rate and rhythm and its electrical activity.

Estrogen: A hormone produced in women by the ovaries
that helps regulate the monthly menstrual cycle.

Exercise stress test: This test is essentially an electrocardiogram that measures your heart rate and its electrical
activity as you exercise on a treadmill or stationary
bicycle. The test is used to detect such heart problems
as angina. It is also useful in determining your level
of physical fitness before launching an exercise program.

Familial hypercholesterolemia (FH): An inherited condition
in which affected people have dangerously high levels
of LDL cholesterol circulating in their bloodstream. The
condition is believed to be caused by a flaw in the gene
that codes for specialized LDL receptors in the liver and
throughout the body, which help clear blood cholesterol
from the bloodstream. There are two forms: *heterozygous FH,* the milder form, in which affected people have
inherited a defective gene from one parent, and *homozygous FH,* a more serious form, in which two defective
genes have been inherited, one from each parent.

Fibric acids: A class of drugs used to lower blood triglyceride levels. The two drugs approved by the U.S. Food
and Drug Administration are *gemfibrozil* and *clofibrate.*

Gene: Part of the nucleus of a cell containing chemical instructions for proteins that make up the human body.

The human body contains between 50,000 and 100,000 genes. Each gene contains the code for producing a single *polypeptide,* the building blocks for proteins. Genes are situated on 23 pairs of *chromosomes* consisting of a long, double strand of DNA *(deoxyribonucleic acid).*

Glucose: A form of sugar that is the major source of energy for every cell in your body.

HMG CoA reductase inhibitors: A new class of drugs that lower blood cholesterol by inhibiting the enzyme *HMG CoA reductase,* which regulates the amount of cholesterol manufactured by the liver. Several of these agents are now being evaluated, including *lovastatin, simvastatin,* and *pravastatin.* So far, only lovastatin has been tested extensively in humans and has been approved by the U.S. Food and Drug Administration for treatment of elevated cholesterol.

Hypertension: A condition in which a person's blood pressure is higher than normal. People with two or more blood pressure readings over 140/90 are considered to have hypertension. People with hypertension are at a greater risk of suffering a heart attack, stroke, or kidney disease. *See also* Blood pressure.

Hypoglycemia: Lower than normal levels of glucose, or sugar, in the blood, often resulting from the administration of too much insulin or sulfonylureas (oral hypoglycemic agents). Symptoms include sweating, shakiness, anxiety, heart palpitations, and weakness. Serious episodes of hypoglycemia may result in confusion, irritability, abnormal behavior, convulsions, coma and, in rare instances, death.

Insulin: A hormone secreted by the pancreas. Insulin helps maintain blood sugar levels. *See also* Diabetes mellitus.

LDL receptors: Specialized areas on the surfaces of cells that attract and bind LDL cholesterol to the cell. About 75 percent of the LDL receptors in your body are located in the liver, where they help clear LDL cholesterol from the bloodstream.

Lipids: A variety of fats that circulate in the bloodstream, including *triglycerides, very low density lipoproteins, low-density lipoproteins,* and *high-density lipoproteins.*

Lipoproteins: Fat and cholesterol that have been packaged along with protein carriers (called *apolipoproteins*) by the liver, thus allowing the fats to circulate in the bloodstream. There are several types of lipoproteins: *very low density lipoproteins* (VLDL), *low-density lipoproteins* (LDL), and *high-density lipoproteins* (HDL).

Lipoprotein (a) or Lp (a): One of numerous protein carriers, or apolipoproteins, that transports fat and cholesterol through the bloodstream. Research suggests that high levels of Lp(a) among people with familial hypercholesterolemia may mean a strong risk of heart attack.

Lipoprotein lipase: An enzyme that helps the body's fat tissues attract and store fats (triglycerides) circulating in the bloodstream.

Monounsaturated fats: *See* Unsaturated fats.

Niacin (nicotinic acid): A B vitamin primarily found in milk, eggs, fish, and poultry, and also in vitamin supplements. A prescription form of niacin is used to lower blood cholesterol.

Nitrates (also known as nitroglycerin): A drug that dilates the coronary arteries and is often prescribed to treat angina pectoris.

Omega-3 fatty acids: A type of polyunsaturated fat that's found mostly in fish and is believed to somehow protect against heart disease.

Partial ileal bypass: A procedure sometimes used to lower blood cholesterol levels by surgically bypassing the part of the intestine responsible for the absorption of cholesterol.

Pedigree: A diagram of a family's ancestors that's used to identify which family members have inherited a particular genetic condition.

Plaque: A buildup of cholesterol and scar tissue on the inner linings of the arteries.

Plasmapheresis: A procedure for lowering blood cholesterol levels by withdrawing a portion of blood plasma from the body, removing some of the LDL cholesterol, and reinjecting the treated blood into the patient.

Plasminogen: A clot-dissolving substance manufactured by the blood vessel wall.

Platelets: Substances that help blood coagulate and form clots.

Polyunsaturated fats: *See* Unsaturated fats.

Probucol: A drug that moderately lowers LDL cholesterol, although no one is sure exactly how it works. Probucol also lowers HDL cholesterol, so it is generally not recommended unless other cholesterol-lowering medications are ineffective. Probucol is an antioxidant that may prevent LDL cholesterol from becoming oxidized, a process in which an oxygen molecule combines with and damages the lipoprotein. Some studies suggest that oxidation of LDL cholesterol within the artery wall may be a critical step in the development of artery-narrowing plaques.

Progesterone: A female sex hormone produced by the ovaries that helps thicken the lining of the uterus each month in preparation for pregnancy. Progesterone also stimulates milk production in a woman's breasts.

Progestin: A synthetic form of progesterone used in birth control pills and postmenopausal hormone replacement therapy.

Saturated fat: A type of fatty acid that's "saturated" with hydrogen atoms. These fats, found in butter, whole milk, ice cream, eggs, red meat, and other animal foods, are solid at room temperature. A diet high in saturated fats is associated with high blood cholesterol levels.

Sodium: A metallic element that, in the body, is responsible for acid-base balance, water balance, nerve transmission, and muscle contraction. Sodium is also a main component of ordinary table salt. A diet high in sodium is associated with high blood pressure in some people.

Soluble fiber: *See* Dietary fiber.

Sulfonylureas: Oral medications, also known as *oral hypoglycemic agents,* given to diabetics to help lower elevated blood sugar levels.

Sympathetic nervous system: Part of the autonomic nervous system that involves such involuntary reflexes as breathing and heart rate.

Systolic blood pressure: *See* Blood pressure.

Thiazide diuretics: One of the most commonly prescribed antihypertensive medications. These drugs work on the kidneys and rid the body of sodium.

Triglycerides: A type of fat that circulates in the bloodstream and is either used for energy or stored in the body's tissues as fat. Triglycerides can be manufactured by the liver and also come from fat in the food we eat.

Unsaturated fats: Fats that are liquid at room temperature and contain double or triple chemical bonds that are easily split. There are two types of unsaturated fats: *polyunsaturated* fats, found in fish, corn, soybean, and safflower oils, have more than one double or triple chemical bond per molecule. *Monounsaturated* fats, found in olive and peanut oils, have only one double or triple chemical bond per molecule. Unsaturated fats are known to help lower blood cholesterol levels.

Xanthomas: Cholesterol deposits that often form on the tendons of people with familial hypercholesterolemia.

Recommended Resources

Contact the following organizations for more information on

Genetic Counseling

National Society of Genetic Counselors
233 Canterbury Drive
Wallingford, PA 19086

More than 1,000 trained genetic counselors throughout the United States are members of this professional organization. Write to the Society for referrals to genetic counselors in your area.

Diabetes

American Diabetes Association
1660 Duke Street
Alexandria, VA 22314
Phone: (800) 232–3472

Call or write for information on the evaluation and treatment of Type I or Type II diabetes.

Diet

American Dietetic Association
National Center for Nutrition and Dietetics
216 West Jackson Boulevard, Suite 800
Chicago, IL 60606–6995

To find a registered dietitian, write to the National Center for Nutrition and Dietetics of the American Dietetic Association and its foundation at the above address.

Heart Disease and Hypertension

American Heart Association
National Center
7320 Greenville Avenue
Dallas, TX 75231

Write the National Center or look in the phone book for the chapter in your area. The American Heart Association has a wealth of materials on low-fat, low-sodium eating, as well as information on how to quit smoking, how to launch an exercise program, and other ways to reduce your risk of heart disease.

National Cholesterol Education Program
Information Center
4733 Bethesda Avenue, Suite 530
Bethesda, MD 20814—4820
Phone: (301) 951—3260

Call or write this branch of the National Institutes of Health for a list of books and pamphlets on high blood cholesterol and advice on how to lower it.

Recommended Reading

Genetics

Bishop, Jerry E., and Michael Waldholz. *Genome*. New York: Simon & Schuster, 1990. The story behind the search for genes that govern human health, illness, and behavior. Includes a chapter on the heritability of heart disease.

Diet

Brody, Jane E. *Jane Brody's Good Food Gourmet*. New York: W. W. Norton & Company, 1990. Savory gourmet recipes you thought you couldn't have on a low-fat diet.
—— *Jane Brody's Good Food Book*. New York: W. W. Norton & Company, 1985. Fact-packed nutrition advice and more than 350 delicious low-fat, low-sodium recipes.
Connor, Sonja L., and William E. Connor. *The New American Diet System*. New York: Simon & Schuster, 1991. A program for lowering the saturated fat and cholesterol in your diet using a single number, the CSI, or Cholesterol-Saturated Fat Index. Includes more than 300 recipes, from snacks to main courses to desserts.

Stress

Eliot, Robert S., and Dennis L. Breo. *Is It Worth Dying For?* New York: Bantam Books, 1984. An excellent description of stress and its effects on your heart, along with solid advice for changing the way you respond to stress.
Friedman, Meyer, and Diane Ulmer. *Treating Type A Behavior and Your Heart*. New York: Alfred A. Knopf, 1984. This best-seller describes Friedman's research on reducing the risk of heart disease through behavior modification. It includes a comprehensive program for recognizing and changing Type A behavior.

Appendixes

Appendix 1: Calories Burned During Common Exercises and Activities

Activity	Calories burned per minute	Activity	Calories burned per minute
Aerobic dancing		Jumping rope	9−12
high-impact	7−10	Racquetball	10−13
low-impact	5−7	Running or jogging	
Badminton (singles)	5−7	12-minute mile	7−10
Basketball	7−10	9-minute mile	10−14
Bicycling		7-minute mile	13−16
5 mph	3−4	5-minute mile	16−21
9 mph	5−7	Sailing	2−3
Bowling	2−3	Sitting quietly	1−2
Calisthenics	3−4	Skating (ice or roller)	4−5
Canoeing (leisure)	2−3	Skiing	
Dancing		downhill	4−6
slow	3−4	cross-country	6−8
fast	5−7	Soccer	5−7
Football	8−10	Squash	11−15
Gardening		Standing quietly	1−2
digging	7−9	Swimming	
hedging	4−5	backstroke	9−12
mowing	6−8	breaststroke	9−12
raking	3−4	crawl stroke	7−9
Golf (walking and		treading water	3−4
carrying bag)	4−6	Tennis	6−8
Hockey	6−7	Volleyball	3−4
Housework		Walking	
cleaning	3−4	3 mph	3−4
ironing	2−4	4 mph	5−6
mopping	3−4	up stairs	7−9
window cleaning	3−4	Weight training	5−7

Appendix 2 : Fat Finder's Guide

Breads, Cereals, Crackers

Food Item	Amount	Calories	Carbohydrates (g)	Total Fat (g)	Saturated Fat (g)	Unsaturated Fat (g)	Cholesterol (mg)	Sodium (mg)
BREADS								
bagel	1	163	30.9	1.4	—	—	—	198
corn bread	1 piece	178	27.5	5.8	1.7	—	—	263
cracked wheat	1 slice	66	12.5	0.9	—	—	—	108
mixed-grain	1 slice	64	11.7	0.9	—	—	—	103
pita pocket	1 pocket	106	20.6	0.6	—	—	—	215
raisin	1 slice	70	13.2	1.0	—	—	—	94
Roman Meal	1 slice	70	13.0	1.0	—	—	—	90
rye	1 slice	66	12.0	0.9	—	—	—	174
pumpernickel	1 slice	82	15.4	0.8	—	—	—	173
white	1 slice	64	11.7	0.9	—	—	—	123
whole-wheat	1 slice	61	11.4	1.1	—	—	—	159
BREAKFAST CEREALS								
corn flakes	1 c	110	25.0	1.0	—	—	—	310
granola	¼ c	127	20.7	4.1	3.0	0.4	0	76
oatmeal								
instant, cooked	¾ c	104	18.1	1.7	—	—	0	286
quick, cooked	¾ c	108	18.9	1.8	0.3	0.7	0	1

Food Item	Amount	Calories	Carbohydrates (g)	Total Fat (g)	Saturated Fat (g)	Unsaturated Fat (g)	Cholesterol (mg)	Sodium (mg)
raisin bran	½ c	86	22.0	0.4	0	0.1	0	178
shredded wheat	1 oz	102	22.6	0.6	—	—	—	3
wheat flakes	1 c	99	22.6	0.5	0.1	0.2	—	270
MUFFINS								
blueberry	1	126	19.5	4.3	—	—	—	200
bran	1	112	16.7	5.1	—	—	—	168
corn	1	130	20.0	1.2	—	—	—	192
English	1	135	26.2	1.1	—	—	0	364
PANCAKES (4-inch size)								
frozen batter	3	210	42.2	1.6	—	—	—	857
from mix	3	180	38.2	1.0	—	—	—	710
frozen	3	246	46.6	3.7	—	—	—	777
WAFFLES								
from mix	1 7-inch	206	27.2	8.0	2.7	—	—	515
frozen	2	190	28.4	6.4	—	—	—	470
PASTA (cooked)								
macaroni	1 c	159	33.7	0.7	—	—	0	1
spaghetti	1 c	159	33.7	0.7	—	—	0	1
CRACKERS								
cheese	5	81	7.8	4.9	—	—	—	180
graham	2	60	11.0	1.0	—	—	—	115

	Serving							
ground wheat	5	70	9.0	3.0	—	—	—	135
Ritz	4	70	9.0	4.0	—	—	—	120
rye	2	45	9.9	0.2	—	—	—	115
Saltines	2	26	4.4	0.6	—	—	—	80
Triscuit	3	60	10.0	2.0	—	—	—	90

Milk, Eggs, and Dairy Products

MILK

	Serving							
whole (3.3%)	8 oz	150	11.4	8.2	5.1	0.3	33	120
low-fat (2%)	8 oz	121	11.7	4.7	2.9	0.2	18	122
low-fat (1%)	8 oz	102	11.7	2.6	1.6	0.1	10	123
skim	8 oz	86	11.9	0.4	0.3	0	4	126
buttermilk	8 oz	99	11.7	2.2	1.3	0	9	257

CREAMS

	Serving							
sour cream	1 tbs	26	0.5	2.5	1.6	0	5	6
half-and-half	1 tbs	20	0.6	1.7	1.1	0	6	6
whipping cream (heavy, fluid)	1 tbs	52	0.4	5.6	3.5	0.2	21	6
whipping cream (pressurized)	1 tbs	8	0.4	0.7	0.4	0	2	4
whipped topping (frozen)	1 tbs	13	0.9	1.0	0.9	0	0	1

NONDAIRY CREAMERS

	Serving							
liquid	½ oz	20	1.7	1.5	0.3	0	0	12
powdered	1 tsp	11	1.1	0.7	0.7	0	0	4

Food Item	Amount	Calories	Carbohydrates (g)	Total Fat (g)	Saturated Fat (g)	Unsaturated Fat (g)	Cholesterol (mg)	Sodium (mg)
YOGURT								
whole	8 oz	139	10.6	7.4	4.8	0.2	29	105
low-fat	8 oz	144	16.0	3.5	2.3	0.1	14	159
skim	8 oz	127	17.4	0.4	0.3	0	4	174
frozen, low-fat	4 oz	100	22	1	—	—	2	60
EGGS								
whole	1 large	75	0.6	5.0	1.6	2.6	213	63
yolk	1 large	59	0.3	5.1	1.6	2.6	213	7
white	1 large	17	0.3	0	—	—	0	55
EGG SUBSTITUTES								
frozen	¼ c	96	1.9	6.7	1.2	3.7	1	120
liquid	1.5 oz	40	0.3	1.6	0.3	0.8	0	33
powdered	.35 oz	44	2.2	1.3	0.4	0.2	57	79
CHEESES								
American	1 oz	106	0.5	8.9	5.6	0.3	27	406
cheddar	1 oz	114	0.4	9.4	6.0	0.3	30	176
cottage cheese								
creamed	1 c	217	5.6	9.5	6.0	0.3	31	850
1% fat	1 c	164	6.2	2.3	1.5	0	10	918
2% fat	1 c	203	8.2	4.4	2.8	0.1	19	918
cream cheese	2 tbs	99	0.8	9.9	6.2	0.4	31	84
monterey jack	1 oz	106	0.2	8.6	—	—	—	152

mozzarella								
whole milk	1 oz	80	0.6	6.1	3.7	0.2	22	106
part skim	1 oz	72	0.8	4.5	2.9	0.1	16	132
ricotta								
whole milk	½ c	216	3.8	16.1	10.3	0.5	63	104
part skim	½ c	171	6.4	9.8	6.1	0.3	38	155
swiss	1 oz	107	1.0	7.8	5.0	0.3	26	74
ICE CREAM								
vanilla								
10% milk fat	½ c	134	15.8	7.5	4.4	0.2	29	58
16% milk fat	½ c	174	16.0	11.8	7.3	0.4	44	54
ice milk	½ c	92	14.5	2.8	1.7	0.2	9	52
sherbet	½ c	135	29.3	1.9	1.2	0	7	44
sorbet	½ c	110	28.0	0.1	—	—	—	9

Meat and Poultry

CHICKEN								
dark meat w skin								
fried	3.5 oz	285	4.1	16.9	4.6	3.9	92	89
roasted	3.5 oz	253	0	15.8	4.4	3.5	91	87
stewed	3.5 oz	233	0	14.7	4.1	3.2	82	70
dark meat w/o skin								
fried	3.5 oz	239	2.6	11.6	3.1	2.8	96	97
roasted	3.5 oz	205	0	9.7	2.7	2.3	93	93
stewed	3.5 oz	192	0	9.0	2.5	2.1	88	74

Food Item	Amount	Calories	Carbohydrates (g)	Total Fat (g)	Saturated Fat (g)	Unsaturated Fat (g)	Cholesterol (mg)	Sodium (mg)
CHICKEN (cont.)								
light meat w skin								
fried	3.5 oz	246	1.8	12.1	3.3	2.7	87	77
roasted	3.5 oz	222	0	10.9	3.1	2.3	84	75
stewed	3.5 oz	201	0	10.0	2.8	2.1	74	63
light meat w/o skin								
fried	3.5 oz	192	0.4	5.5	1.5	1.3	90	81
roasted	3.5 oz	173	0	4.5	1.3	1.0	85	77
stewed	3.5 oz	159	0	4.0	1.1	0.9	77	65
TURKEY (ROASTED)								
dark meat								
w skin	3.5 oz	221	0	11.5	3.5	3.1	89	76
w/o skin	3.5 oz	187	0	7.2	2.4	2.2	85	79
light meat								
w skin	3.5 oz	197	0	8.3	2.3	2.0	76	63
w/o skin	3.5 oz	157	0	3.2	1.0	0.9	69	64
ground turkey	3.5 oz	225	0	14.0	4.5	3.2	92	74
BEEF								
brisket, braised								
with fat	3.5 oz	391	0	32.4	13.2	1.2	93	61
fat removed	3.5 oz	241	0	12.8	4.6	0.4	93	72

chuck arm potroast, braised								
with fat	3.5 oz	350	0	26.0	10.7	1.0	99	60
fat trimmed	3.5 oz	231	0	10	3.8	0.4	101	66
chuck blade roast, braised								
with fat	3.5 oz	383	0	30.4	12.7	1.1	103	63
fat trimmed	3.5 oz	270	0	15.3	6.2	0.5	106	71
flank steak, broiled								
with fat	3.5 oz	254	0	16.3	7.0	0.5	71	82
fat trimmed	3.5 oz	243	0	15.0	6.4	0.5	70	83
ground beef, pan fried								
extra lean	3.5 oz	255	0	16.4	6.5	0.6	81	70
lean	3.5 oz	275	0	19.1	7.5	0.7	84	77
regular	3.5 oz	306	0	22.6	8.9	0.8	89	84
eye of round, roasted								
with fat	3.5 oz	243	0	14.2	5.8	0.5	73	59
fat trimmed	3.5 oz	183	0	6.5	2.5	0.2	69	62
sirloin steak, broiled								
with fat	3.5 oz	280	0	18.0	7.5	0.7	90	63
fat trimmed	3.5 oz	208	0	8.7	3.6	0.4	89	66
PORK								
bacon								
broiled/fried	3 pieces	109	0.1	9.4	3.3	1.1	16	303
center loin, with fat								
broiled	3.5 oz	316	0	22.1	8.0	2.5	97	70
pan fried	3.5 oz	375	0	30.5	11.0	3.5	103	72
roasted	3.5 oz	305	0	21.8	7.9	2.5	91	64

Food Item	Amount	Calories	Carbohydrates (g)	Total Fat (g)	Saturated Fat (g)	Unsaturated Fat (g)	Cholesterol (mg)	Sodium (mg)
PORK (*cont.*)								
center loin, fat trimmed								
broiled	3.5 oz	231	0	10.5	3.6	1.3	98	78
pan fried	3.5 oz	266	0	15.9	5.5	2.0	107	85
roasted	3.5 oz	240	0	13.1	4.5	1.6	91	69
ham, cured								
canned, lean	3.5 oz	120	0	4.6	1.5	0.4	38	1,255
canned, regular	3.5 oz	190	0	13.0	4.3	1.5	39	1,240
sausage links	1 link	48	0.1	4.1	1.4	0.5	11	168
sausage patties	1 patty	100	0.3	8.4	2.9	1.0	22	349
VEAL								
chuck (braised/roasted/ stewed)	3 oz	200	0	10.9	5.2	—	—	41
loin (broiled)	3 oz	199	0	11.4	5.5	—	—	55
rib roast	3 oz.	229	0	14.4	6.9	—	—	57
ORGAN MEATS								
chicken liver	3.5 oz	157	0.9	5.5	1.8	0.9	631	51
beef liver	3.5 oz	161	3.4	4.9	1.9	1.1	389	70
beef tongue	3.5 oz	283	0.3	20.7	8.9	0.8	107	60

LUNCHEON MEATS

bologna								
beef	1 slice	72	0.2	6.6	2.8	0.3	13	226
turkey	1 slice	60	0.6	4.5	1.4	1.1	20	222
chicken roll	2 slices	90	1.4	4.2	1.2	0.9	28	331
corned beef	1 oz	43	0	1.7	0.7	0.1	13	270
frankfurters								
beef	1	180	1.0	16.3	6.9	0.8	35	585
beef and pork	1	144	1.2	13.1	4.8	1.2	22	504
chicken	1	116	3.1	8.8	2.5	1.8	45	617
turkey	1	100	0.6	8.1	2.7	2.1	39	472
ham								
lean, 5% fat	1 slice	37	0.3	1.4	0.5	0.1	13	405
regular, 11% fat	1 slice	52	0.9	3.0	1.0	0.3	13	373
pastrami	1 oz	99	0.9	8.3	3.0	0.3	26	348
turkey breast	1 slice	23	0	0.3	0.1	0.1	9	301

Fish and Shellfish

FISH

bass, baked	4 oz	287	3.0	19.4	—	—	—	68
cod, baked	3 oz	89	0	0.7	0.1	0.2	47	66
fish filets								
(frozen, batter-dipped)	3 oz	180	15.0	10	—	—	—	230
flounder, baked	3.5 oz	202	0	8.2	0.1	—	—	237

Food Item	Amount	Calories	Carbohydrates (g)	Total Fat (g)	Saturated Fat (g)	Unsaturated Fat (g)	Cholesterol (mg)	Sodium (mg)
FISH (*cont.*)								
grouper, baked	3 oz	100	0	1.1	0.3	0.3	40	45
haddock, baked	3 oz	95	0	0.8	0.1	0.3	63	74
halibut, baked	3 oz	119	0	2.5	0.4	0.8	35	59
mackerel, baked	3 oz	223	0	15.1	3.6	3.7	64	71
ocean perch, baked	3 oz	103	0	1.8	0.3	0.5	46	82
salmon, pink canned	3 oz	118	0	5.1	1.3	1.7	—	471
sardines, in oil	2	50	0	2.8	0.4	1.2	34	121
snapper, baked	3 oz	109	0	1.5	0.3	0.5	40	48
sole, filet	1	80	0.6	0.8	—	—	—	162
trout, baked	3 oz.	129	0	3.7	0.7	1.3	62	29
tuna fish								
canned in oil	3 oz	169	0	7.0	1.3	2.5	15	301
water packed	3 oz	111	0	0.4	0.1	0.1	15	303
SHELLFISH								
clams, steamed	3 oz	126	4.4	1.7	0.2	0.5	57	95
crab, steamed	3 oz.	87	0	1.5	—	—	—	237
crab cakes	1 cake	93	0.3	4.5	0.9	1.4	90	198
lobster, steamed	3 oz	83	1.1	0.5	0.1	0.1	61	323
mussels, steamed	3 oz	147	6.3	3.8	0.7	1.0	48	313

Food	Serving							
oysters, steamed	3 oz	117	6.7	4.2	1.1	1.3	96	190
scallops								
breaded, fried	2 large	67	3.1	3.4	0.8	0.9	19	144
shrimp								
steamed	3 oz	84	0	0.9	0.2	0.4	166	190
breaded, fried	3 oz	206	9.8	10.4	1.8	4.3	150	292
Fruits and Vegetables								
apples	1 med	81	21.1	0.1	0.1	0.1	0	1
apricots	3 med	51	11.8	0.4	0	0.1	0	1
bananas	1 med	105	26.7	0.6	0.2	0.1	0	1
blueberries	1 c	82	20.5	0.6	—	—	0	9
cantaloupe	1 c	57	13.4	0.4	—	—	0	14
cherries	10 med	49	11.3	0.7	0.1	0.2	0	0
dates (dried)	10	228	61.0	0.4	—	—	0	2
fruit cocktail								
in heavy syrup	½ c	93	24.2	0.1	0	0	0	7
in juice	½ c	56	14.7	0	0	0	0	4
grapefruit								
pink	½ med	37	9.5	0.1	0	0	0	0
white	½ med	39	9.9	0.1	0	0	0	0
grapes	1 c	58	15.8	0.3	0.1	0.1	0	2
oranges	1 med	59	14.4	0.4	0	0.1	0	0
peaches								
raw	1 med	37	9.7	0.1	0	0	0	0

Food Item	Amount	Calories	Carbohydrates (g)	Total Fat (g)	Saturated Fat (g)	Unsaturated Fat (g)	Cholesterol (mg)	Sodium (mg)
peaches (*cont.*)								
canned, syrup	1 c	190	51.0	0.3	0	0.1	0	16
canned, juice	1 c	109	28.7	0.1	0	0	0	11
pears								
raw	1 med	98	25.1	0.7	0	0.2	0	1
canned, syrup	1 c	188	48.9	0.3	0	0.1	0	13
canned, juice	1 c	123	32.1	0.2	0	0	0	10
pineapple								
raw	1 c	77	19.2	0.7	0	0.2	0	1
canned, syrup	1 c	199	51.5	0.3	0	0.1	0	3
canned, juice	1 c	150	39.2	0.2	0	0.1	0	4
plums	1 med	36	8.6	0.4	0	0.1	0	0
prunes								
canned, syrup	5	90	23.9	0.2	0	0	0	2
dried	5	100	26.3	0.2	0	0	0	1
raisins	⅔ c	300	79.1	0.5	0.2	0.1	0	12
strawberries								
raw	1 c	45	10.5	0.6	0	0.3	0	2
frozen, sweet	1 c	245	66.1	0.3	0	0.2	0	8
frozen, unsweet	1 c	52	13.6	0.2	0	0.1	0	3

watermelon	1 c	50	11.5	0.7	—	—	0	33
asparagus								
fresh, boiled	½ c	22	4.0	0.3	0.1	0.1	0	4
canned	½ c	24	3.0	0.8	0.2	0.3	0	—
avocado, raw								
California	1 med	306	12.0	30	4.5	3.5	0	21
Florida	1 med	339	27.1	27.0	5.3	4.5	0	14
baked beans								
vegetarian	1 c	235	52.1	1.1	0.3	0.5	0	1,008
w pork	1 c	247	49.1	2.6	1.0	0.3	17	1,113
beets								
fresh, boiled	½ c	26	5.7	0	0	0	0	42
canned	½ c	27	6.1	0.1	0	0	0	—
pickled	½ c	75	18.6	0.1	0	0	0	301
broccoli								
raw, chopped	½ c	12	2.3	0.2	0	0.1	0	12
boiled	½ c	23	4.3	0.2	0	0.1	0	8
frozen	½ c	25	4.9	0.1	0	0.1	0	22
brussels sprouts								
fresh, boiled	½ c	30	6.8	0.4	0.1	0.2	0	17
frozen	½ c	33	6.5	0.3	0.1	0.2	0	18
cabbage								
green	½ c	8	1.9	0.1	0	0	0	6

Food Item	Amount	Calories	Carbohydrates (g)	Total Fat (g)	Saturated Fat (g)	Unsaturated Fat (g)	Cholesterol (mg)	Sodium (mg)
cabbage (*cont.*)								
red	½ c	10	2.1	0.1	0	0	0	4
coleslaw	½ c	42	7.5	1.6	0.2	0.8	5	14
carrots								
raw	1 med	31	7.3	0.1	0	0.1	0	25
canned	½ c	17	4.0	0.1	0	0.1	0	176
frozen	½ c	26	6.0	0.1	0	0	0	43
cauliflower								
raw	½ c	12	2.5	0.1	0	0	0	7
boiled	½ c	15	2.9	0.1	0	0.1	0	4
frozen	½ c	17	3.4	0.2	0	0.1	0	16
celery	1 stalk	6	1.5	0.1	0	0	0	35
chickpeas								
boiled	1 c	269	45.0	4.3	0.4	1.9	0	11
canned	1 c	285	54.3	2.7	0.3	1.2	0	413
corn								
fresh, boiled	½ c	89	20.6	1.1	0.2	0.5	0	14
canned	½ c	66	15.2	0.8	0.1	0.4	0	—
cream style	½ c	93	23.2	0.5	0.1	0.3	0	365
frozen	½ c	67	16.8	0.1	0	0	0	4

cucumber, raw	½ c	7	1.5	0.1	0	0	0	1
green beans								
fresh, boiled	½ c	22	4.9	0.2	0	0.1	0	2
canned	½ c	13	3.1	0.1	0	0	0	170
frozen	½ c	18	4.2	0.1	0	0	0	9
kidney beans								
boiled	1 c	225	40.4	0.9	0.1	0.5	0	4
canned	1 c	208	38.1	0.8	0.1	0.4	0	889
lentils, boiled	1 c	231	39.9	0.7	0.1	0.3	0	4
lettuce								
Romaine	½ c	4	0.7	0.1	0	0	0	2
Iceberg	½ c	3	0.4	0	0	0	0	2
lima beans								
fresh, boiled	1 c	217	39.3	0.7	0.2	0.3	0	4
canned	1 c	191	35.9	0.4	0.1	0.2	0	809
mixed vegetables								
canned	½ c	39	7.6	0.2	0	0.1	0	122
frozen	½ c	54	11.9	0.1	0	0.1	0	32
mushrooms								
raw	½ c	9	1.6	0.2	0	0.1	0	1
fresh, boiled	½ c	21	4.0	0.4	0	0.1	0	2
canned	½ c	19	3.9	0.2	0	0.1	0	—
onions								
raw	½ c	27	5.9	0.2	0	0.1	0	2

Food Item	Amount	Calories	Carbohydrates (g)	Total Fat (g)	Saturated Fat (g)	Unsaturated Fat (g)	Cholesterol (mg)	Sodium (mg)
onions (*cont.*)								
cooked	½ c	29	6.6	0.2	0	0.1	0	8
peas, green								
boiled	½ c	67	12.5	0.2	0	0.1	0	2
canned	½ c	59	10.7	0.3	0.1	0.1	0	186
frozen	½ c	63	11.4	0.2	0	0.1	0	70
peas, split								
boiled	1 c	231	41.4	0.8	0.1	0.3	0	4
peppers, sweet	½ c	12	2.7	0.2	0	0.1	0	2
pinto beans								
boiled	1 c	235	43.9	0.9	0.2	0.3	0	3
canned	1 c	186	34.9	0.8	0.2	0.3	0	998
potatoes								
baked w skin	1	220	51.0	0.2	0.1	0.1	0	16
baked w/o skin	1	145	33.6	0.2	0	0.1	0	8
boiled w/o skin	1	116	27.0	0.1	0	0.1	0	7
canned w/o skin	½ c	54	12.3	0.2	0	0.1	0	—
french fries	10	158	20	8.3	2.5	3.8	0	108
hash browns	½ c	163	16.6	10.9	4.2	1.3	—	19
mashed, flakes	½ c	118	15.8	5.9	3.6	0.3	15	349

mashed, homemade	½ c	111	17.5	4.4	1.1	1.3	2	309
potato salad	½ c	179	14.0	10.3	1.8	4.7	86	661
au gratin	½ c	160	13.7	9.3	5.8	0.3	29	528
scalloped	½ c	105	13.2	4.5	2.8	0.2	14	409
rice								
white, cooked	½ c	111	24.8	0.1	—	—	0	0
instant, cooked	1 c	90	19.9	0	—	—	0	0
fried	½ c	159	25.2	4.8	0.7	1.8	0	551
spinach								
raw	½ c	6	1.0	0.1	0	0	0	22
boiled	½ c	21	3.4	0.2	0	0.1	0	63
canned	½ c	25	3.6	0.5	0.1	0.2	0	29
frozen	½ c	27	5.1	0.2	0	0.1	0	82
squash, summer								
raw	½ c	13	2.8	0.1	0	0.1	0	1
boiled	½ c	18	3.9	0.3	0.1	0.1	0	1
squash, winter								
baked	½ c	39	8.9	0.6	0.1	0.3	0	1
sweet potatoes								
baked	1 med	118	27.7	0.1	0	0.1	0	12
boiled	½ c	172	39.8	0.5	0.1	0.2	0	21
canned, syrup	½ c	106	24.9	0.3	0.1	0.1	0	38
tomatoes								
raw	1 med	24	5.3	0.3	0	0.1	0	10
stewed	½ c	34	8.3	0.2	0	0.1	0	325

Index